SPEECH THERAPY
AND ENT SURGERY

SPEECH THERAPY AND ENT SURGERY

T R Bull MB BS(Lond) FRCS(Eng)

Consultant Surgeon, Royal National Throat,
Nose & Ear Hospital, and Metropolitan Ear,
Nose & Throat Hospital, London

Hon. Lecturer, Institute of Laryngology &
Otology, London

Lecturer, National Hospitals College of
Speech Sciences, London

Joyce L Cook MCST

Senior Speech Therapist, Royal National Throat,
Nose & Ear Hospital, London

BLACKWELL SCIENTIFIC PUBLICATIONS
OXFORD LONDON EDINBURGH MELBOURNE

© 1976 Blackwell Scientific Publications
Osney Mead, Oxford OX2 0EL
85 Marylebone High Street, London W1M 3DE
9 Forrest Road, Edinburgh EH1 2QH
P.O. Box 9, North Balwyn, Victoria, Australia

ISBN 0 632 09410 9

First published 1976

Distributed in the U.S.A. by
J.B. Lippincott Company, Philadelphia
and in Canada by
J.B. Lippincott Company of Canada Ltd, Toronto

Set in Monotype Times

Printed in Great Britain by
Burgess & Son (Abingdon) Ltd, Station Road, Abingdon, Oxfordshire

CONTENTS

PREFACE

This book aims to cover the specialist field where the roles of the Ear, Nose and Throat Surgeon and the Speech Therapist overlap. The scope of speech therapy is broad, covering the many aspects of speech, voice and language. The speech therapist may be involved in one or several of these aspects. This book is concerned specifically with those voice disorders which present in an ENT department, and which may subsequently be referred to the speech therapist.

Speech therapy for congenital and acquired central nervous system disorders and congenital deafness is not dealt with in this book, and the cleft palate problem is also not included. Cleft palate surgery is mainly handled by the plastic surgeon, and the trend is for congenital central speech problems to be managed at special centres. The anatomy has been confined to the head and neck and emphasizes clinical aspects.

It is helpful if the speech therapist is aware of those conditions in the ENT field which she can help, and is equally alert to those where speech therapy has no part to play. It is important in treating disorders of the voice that there is referral back to the ENT surgeon by the speech therapist so the case can be discussed and for the larynx to be kept under observation by the surgeon. The speech therapist may also have further information to offer, following the case history and assessment of the voice. It is important that speech therapy is not undertaken until an ENT opinion has been obtained. The speech therapist must know the condition of the larynx and upper respiratory tract before correct treatment can be planned. It should be remembered that voice disorders may be seen in a child with a speech and language problem, and if there is considerable difficulty in understanding the child's speech a defect of voice due to laryngeal abnormality may be missed if the speech therapist does not ensure an ENT opinion.

The reorganization of the Health Service and the formation of an integrated speech therapy service has meant that a number of speech therapists, who have worked mainly with children within the school health service, may now be called upon to treat a wider range of patients, including adults.

We hope that this book will help speech therapists in the ear, nose and throat aspects of their work.

T R Bull   *London, 1976*

Joyce Cook

CHAPTER ONE
CLINICAL ANATOMY

THE NECK

Many of the important structures in the neck are apparent on surface examination. The anatomy that is visible depends on the amount of subcutaneous fat but many structures that cannot be seen can be palpated. The most obvious mid-line laryngeal structure is the Adam's apple which is the prominence of the thyroid cartilage. This cartilage is so-called because it is shaped like and acts as a shield* to the larynx. There is a notch which can be felt in the mid-line superiorly and the two cornua extend laterally on each side from the notch. The angle at which the alae of the thyroid cartilage meet anteriorly is more acute in the male thus the thyroid cartilage is more prominent. Above the thyroid cartilage and attached to it by the thyrohyoid membrane and muscle, is the hyoid bone. The hard body of the bone can be felt in the mid-line with the cornua extending laterally.

Below the thyroid cartilage, a depression can be felt in the mid-line which is the cricothyroid membrane and below this is the firm complete ring of the cricoid cartilage. The rings of the trachea may be seen in a thin person and can be felt extending to the suprasternal notch, bounded by the medial ends of the clavicles and the superior border of the manubrium sternum. Unlike the cricoid, the trachea can be compressed because the cartilage rings supporting the trachea are deficient posteriorly and bridged by fibrous tissue. The hyoid, thyroid and cricoid are all mobile and move up and down on swallowing. Superiorly, the hyoid gives attachment to the muscles of the base of the tongue and inferiorly, the hyoid and thyroid are attached to the manubrium sternum

* Thureos—shield

1

by the sternothyroid and sternohyoid muscles. These flat muscles are sometimes called the strap muscles; the muscles attached externally to the larynx are known as the extrinsic muscles and these raise and lower the larynx, whereas the intrinsic muscles control vocal cord movement. A 'creaking' sensation known as crepitus is apparent on moving the larynx with the hands, this normal characteristic is lost when extensive cancer involves the larynx.

The *neck muscles* which are most obvious anteriorly are the sternomastoids. These two powerful muscles extend from the mastoid processes and occipital bones of the base of the skull to the sternum and clavicles, and are made obvious if the forehead is pressed against the palm of the hand. The anterior border ends in the firm round fibrous head which can be seen and felt and is the muscles' medial attachment to the manubrium. The small inferior belly of the omohyoid can sometimes be seen emerging from the posterior border of the sternomastoid muscle to its attachment to the scapula. The strap muscles of the larynx are thin, flat muscles running vertically from the hyoid and thyroid superficial to the thyroid gland to be attached to the manubrium sternum. They are not obvious in the neck, on examination or palpation.

The *carotid artery* pulsation may be seen in the neck and is usually most obvious at the point of division of the internal and external carotid vessels, the bulb of the carotid, which lies lateral to the thyroid cartilage. The pulsation of the carotid artery can be felt between the thyroid cartilage and the anterior border of the sternomastoid muscle.

The main *lymph nodes* in the neck are the deep cervical lymph nodes. These lie along the course of the internal jugular vein which accompanies the carotid artery within the fascia of the carotid sheath. Small soft, mobile lymph nodes may be palpable in a normal neck. The tonsillar node which is one of the superior deep cervical nodes is usually palpable near the angle of the mandible, particularly in children who have larger and more extensive lymph nodes than adults. In inflammatory disease of the head and neck and upper respiratory tract, the lymph nodes are enlarged, soft and tender. In acute tonsillitis therefore, the tonsillar nodes may be visibly enlarged and are always palpable. In malignant disease, the cancer may spread to the lymph nodes, which become large, irregular and hard, but usually not tender and painful, unless the nodes are infected or the trunks of the nerves of the brachial or cervical plexus underlying the node are invaded.

Thyroid Gland

The two lobes of the thyroid gland lie on either side of the larynx joined across the mid-line by the isthmus. The gland may vary in size from time to time, particularly in women when it may enlarge prior to menstruation. In a thin neck the outline of a normal thyroid can be seen. The gland can be palpated and it is easier to feel the thyroid gland when standing behind the patient for the examiner's hands take up the shape of the neck. The thyroid gland is attached by fascia to the thyroid, cricoid and trachea and moves up and down with the larynx on swallowing.

The thyroid gland is an endocrine organ similar to the pituitary, ovary and adrenals, and produces several hormones including thyroxine. The production of thyroxine is under control of the thyrotrophic hormone of the pituitary. Thyroxine affects the rate of metabolism of the body; if the production is normal, a person is known as euthyroid.

In *hyperthyroidism*, an excess of thyroxine is released and results in thyrotoxicosis (Graves' disease). This condition is characterized by a hyperactive, restless person, with hot, sweaty skin, particularly on the palms, and a rapid, large-volumed pulse. A large appetite is associated with a thin body, and a fine tremor is noticeable when the hands are outstretched. Changes in the eye occur, and the white sclera of the eye may be apparent all around the iris; the lids are retracted and the eye also may become prominent (exophthalmos) causing a staring appearance. In severe cases, the eye is markedly pushed forward, making it impossible to close the lids and ulceration of the cornea may result. Hyperthyroidism may be associated with a diffuse enlargement of the gland so that a thyroid swelling or goitre may be seen. The condition may be treated medically, but surgical removal of part of the overactive thyroid lobes is often necessary— partial thyroidectomy. In operations on the thyroid gland, the recurrent laryngeal nerves are at risk and care is taken to preserve them. Surgical damage to one nerve, or involvement of the nerve by a thyroid cancer, results in hoarseness from paralysis of the vocal cord on that side. If both nerves are damaged, the cords lie immobile near the mid-line and severely limit the airway.

In *hypothyroidism* the production of thyroxine is below normal. This results in a slow, overweight person with a dry skin and a slow pulse; there is a yellow complexion and thin, atrophic hair; the condition is known as myxoedema. There is a dislike of cold weather, whereas in hyperthyroidism hot weather is found to be uncomfortable. A thickening of the vocal cords and ventricular bands is seen in myxoedema and causes hoarseness which may be the presenting symptom and can be misdiagnosed as chronic laryngitis. Children may be born with absent or diminished thyroid function, which produces a characteristic form of retardation known as cretinism. Early detection of this condition and treatment with a thyroxine-like preparation is important for normal or near-normal development to occur.

UPPER RESPIRATORY TRACT

The Nose

The nasal cavity extends horizontally from the vestibule of the nose to the postnasal space where the soft palate separates it from the oropharynx. The vestibule of the nose faces inferiorly but if the tip of the nose is elevated with the thumb or with a nasal speculum, the posterior direction of the nasal cavity is apparent. The nasal septum which divides the nasal cavity into two nasal fossae, is normally straight but may, as a result of trauma, be deviated and cause airway obstruction. The inferior turbinates are the most obvious structure seen anteriorly in the nose and the red swelling on the lateral wall of the nose may be prominent and can be mistaken for a nasal polyp or tumour. The middle and superior turbinates are not visible without good lighting and a nasal speculum. The turbinates are finger-like projections from the lateral wall of the nose and extend to the postnasal space. The mucous membrane of the nose and upper respiratory tract is ciliated, columnar epithelium. The membrane is covered with a film of mucus and ciliary movement in the posterior direction ensures that a constant film of mucus moves towards the postnasal space. Any particles inhaled are carried to the back of the nose in this mucus which is then swallowed. Excess nasal mucus may be produced in dusty and irritant environments or from cigarettes, or in those people with a sensitive or allergic nasal mucous membrane (*e.g.* chronic rhinitis or hay fever). The increase in mucus passing from the postnasal space into the oropharynx may cause the irritating but usually minor symptom often called 'postnasal drip'. Normally, one is unaware of the passage of this mucus.

The *postnasal space* is occupied in children by lymphoid tissue called the adenoid. This tissue has normally regressed by puberty and it is rare for adenoids to persist into adult life. In children, large adenoids may cause obstruction of the nose and may also interfere with the function of the Eustachian tube, which links the middle ear to the postnasal space, for the orifice of the tube is closely related to the adenoids. The postnasal space is concealed from view and can be seen with a small, angled mirror placed in the oropharynx posterior to the soft palate (Figure 1). In adults, a good view is usually obtained, but in children, the gag reflex and fear of instruments usually only allows a glimpse of this region. A lateral X-ray, however, is a helpful investigation, showing the soft tissue shadow of the adenoids and giving a reliable indication of their size, and the degree of obstruction they may be causing to the postnasal space (Figure 2).

The Pharynx

The *tongue* is a muscular organ supplied by the XIIth cranial nerve, the hypoglossal nerve. The intrinsic muscles, consisting of transverse and vertical fibres, alter the shape of

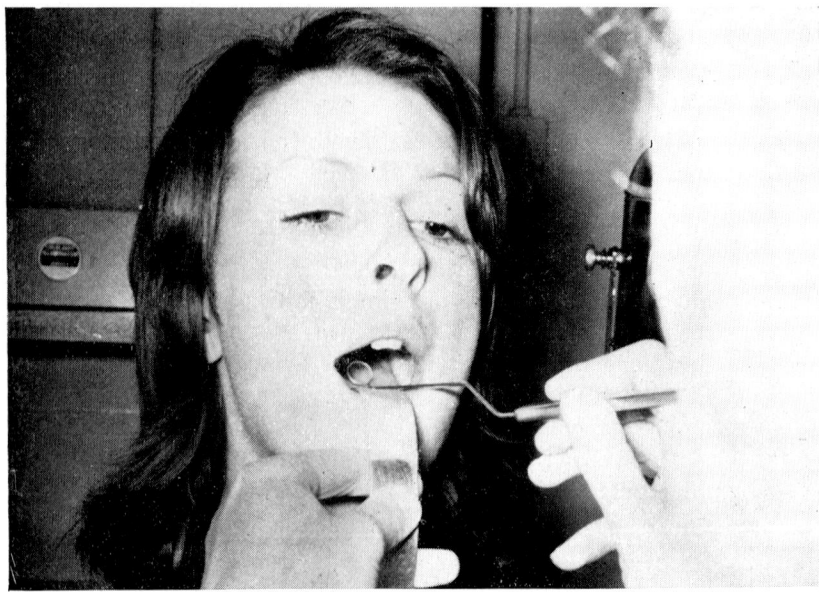

Figure 1 Examination of postnasal space.

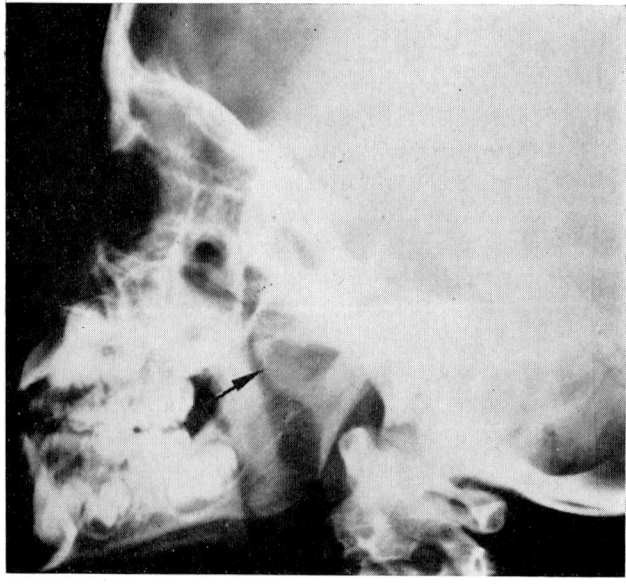

Figure 2 Lateral skull X-ray of a child to show the soft tissue swelling of the adenoids (arrowed). The adenoids in this case are large, limiting the airway, but there is not complete occlusion of the postnasal space.

the tongue and the position is controlled by the extrinsic muscles with attachment to the mandible (genioglossus), hyoid bone (hyoglossus), palate (palatoglossus) and base of skull (styloglossus—attached to the styloid process). The frenulum linguae is a fibrous band attached to the under surface of the tongue anteriorly. This is usually a structure of no clinical significance but the fibrous tissue may extend to the tip of the tongue and be a short, tight band limiting protrusion and movement of the tongue.

On the surface of the tongue there are the small, red, fungiform papillae, these are more numerous and obvious in children. On these papillae the taste buds are concentrated. The circumvallate taste papillae are obvious on the posterior third of the tongue (Figure 3) and when particularly prominent may be mistaken by the patient for cancer.

The most obvious structures in the oropharynx are the tonsils and uvula. The uvula serves no particular function

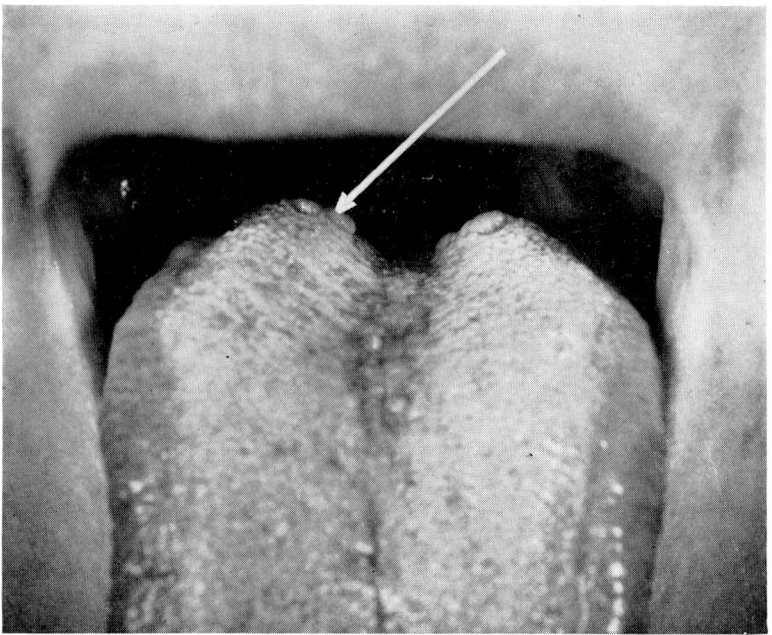

Figure 3 Circumvallate taste papillae on the base of the tongue are often prominent, and may be mistaken by a patient for serious disease.

and is rarely the cause of symptoms although a retention cyst or particularly long uvula may cause irritation and require removal. The uvula is not uncommonly bifid; this is a minor congenital deformity with no symptoms (Figure 4). This abnormality is of importance, however, as it may be associated with a submucous palatal cleft, which is to be detected by observation and palpation of the hard palate.

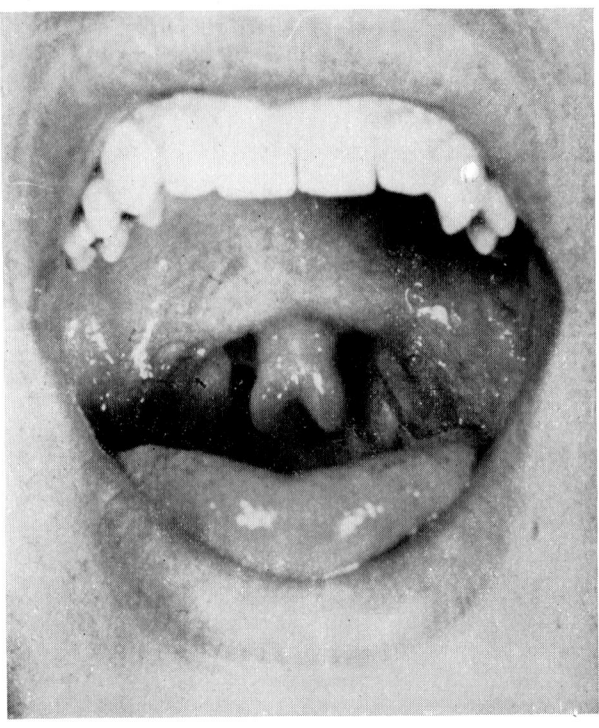

Figure 4 Bifid uvula. This is a not uncommon chance finding on routine examination. It may be associated with a submucous palatal cleft.

The tonsils are collections of lymphoid tissue placed in the tonsillar fossae limited by the fauces or pillars; the anterior pillar is the palatoglossus muscle, and posteriorly is the palatopharyngeus muscle which is one of the longitudinal muscles of the pharynx extending from the palate to be attached to the posterior border of the alae of the thyroid cartilage. The tip of the epiglottis is not infrequently visible on full protrusion of the tongue.

The *larynx* like the postnasal space is examined with a mirror. A clear view of the base of the tongue, epiglottis, valleculae, arytenoids, ventricular bands, vocal cords and pyriform fossae can be obtained. In children, it is difficult or impossible to see this anatomy. Not only is the gag reflex and full cooperation a problem, but the epiglottis in a child is very curved, the so-called infantile epiglottis, and the prominent curve posteriorly obscures a clear view of the vocal cords. The anatomy of the larynx seen on direct laryngoscopy is illustrated in Figure 5. The cord movement on phonation can be seen, as well as any lesion affecting the various structures.

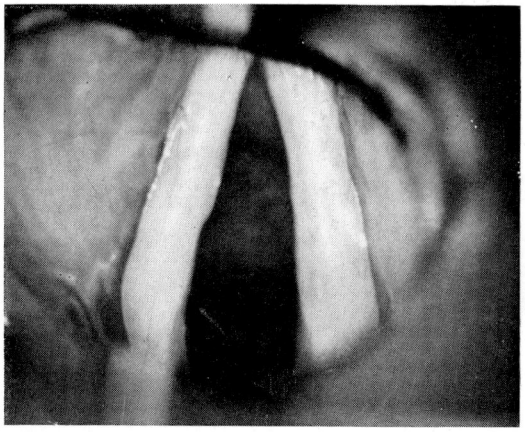

Figure 5   Normal vocal cords seen on direct microlaryngoscopy.

The vocal cords are attached anteriorly to the thyroid cartilage at the angle where the alae meet. The posterior ends of the cords are attached to the arytenoid cartilages. This pair of cartilages articulate with the cricoid cartilage and it is the muscles which are attached to the arytenoid that move this cartilage at the cricoarytenoid joint and alter the position of the vocal cord. The cricoarytenoid joint is sometimes involved in rheumatoid arthritis with limitation of movement. There are two pairs of small unimportant cartilages (the corniculate and cuneiform cartilages) placed on the superior surface of the arytenoids. The lateral prominence of the arytenoid is a muscular process to which the important intrinsic muscles of the larynx, controlling vocal cord movement, are attached. The vocal cord is attached to the anterior vocal process of the arytenoid. There are a number of small muscles acting on the cricoarytenoid joint.

The posterior cricoarytenoid muscles arise from the posterior aspect of the cricoid cartilage and rotate the arytenoids outwards so that the cords move laterally. These muscles, therefore, control the movement of cord abduction; they are the most important muscles in the larynx and perhaps in the whole body, for it is these muscles which 'open' the vocal cords ensuring the airway. The posterior cricoarytenoid muscle is supplied by the recurrent laryngeal nerve and damage to this nerve results in a failure of cord abduction so that the cord lies immobile near the mid-line.

The lateral cricoarytenoid muscle arises from the superior margin of the cricoid cartilage and is attached to the anterior border of the muscular process of the arytenoid. The muscle rotates the arytenoid inwards causing adduction of the cord; the lateral fibres, however, may well, because of their angle, be responsible in part for abduction of the cord as well. The lateral and posterior cricoarytenoid muscles evidently work together to rotate the arytenoid and control adduction and abduction of the cord. The transverse arytenoid muscle

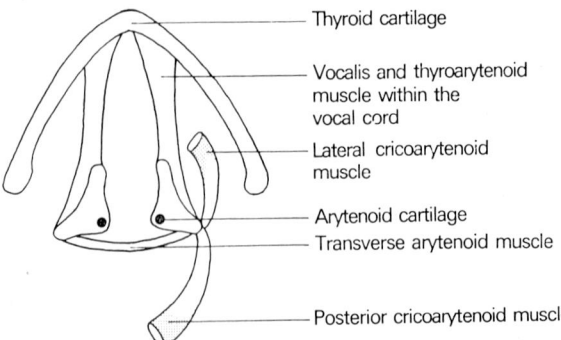

Figure 6   Horizontal section of the larynx to show muscles.

connects the arytenoids and contraction approximates the cartilages causing adduction.

The other intrinsic muscles to the larynx are the vocalis within the vocal cord and the thyroarytenoid muscle arising from the angle of the thyroid cartilage and adjacent alae. The vocalis is in fact a part of the thyroarytenoid, and these muscles control the length and tension of the vocal cord. The remaining intrinsic laryngeal muscle is the cricothyroid muscle which is concerned in control of the length of the vocal cord. All the intrinsic muscles acting on the vocal cord are supplied by the recurrent laryngeal nerve. This branch of the vagus is, therefore, the critical motor supply for the larynx and damage results in cord immobility; the nerve also supplies sensation to the mucous membrane of the trachea and larynx up to the vocal cords.

An important muscle which is not concerned with vocal cord movement but which is attached to the cricoid cartilage posteriorly is the cricopharyngeus. The fibres of this muscle encircle the opening of the oesophagus and are involved in the swallowing reflex. Abnormal contraction of this muscle causes symptoms and the muscle is of importance after laryngectomy in helping to control air expulsion when pseudo-voice is developed.

X-rays help to show the anatomy of the larynx. A lateral X-ray of the neck will show the outline of the soft tissue structures of the pharynx, larynx and trachea and also demonstrate the air-filled spaces. A simple lateral and antero-posterior X-ray may assist in localizing fairly gross abnormalities, such as narrowing or widening of the laryngeal inlet, upper trachea or upper oesophagus and are used as preliminary investigations. Tomograms, however, are more elaborate X-rays and are helpful in demonstrating changes in anatomy caused by laryngeal disease. They are a series of X-rays taken at consecutive depths of 'cuts' through a structure and a laryngeal tomogram demonstrates the cords, ventricles, ventricular bands and upper trachea. A small abnormality is apparent in this type of X-ray. The laryngogram is an X-ray in which the surface of the laryngeal mucosa is covered with a radioopaque substance (Figure 7). Although the anatomy is well demonstrated, it is an unpleasant test for the patient and requires skill to obtain good pictures. Good tomograms have tended to displace the laryngogram as an investigation.

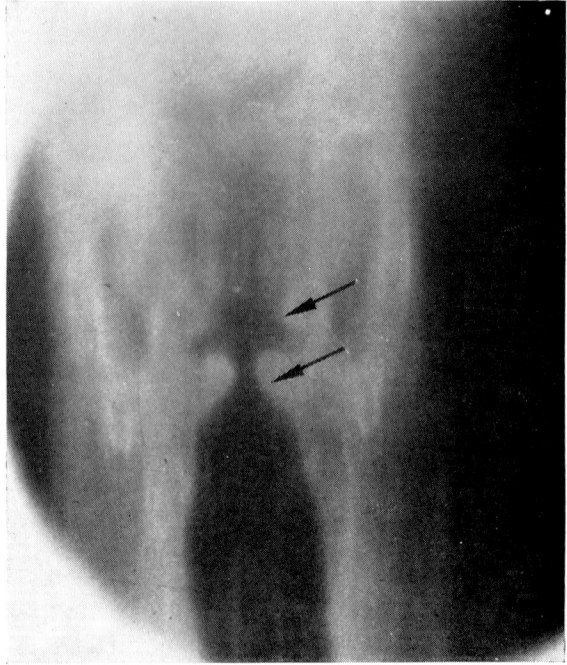

Figure 7   Laryngeal tomogram X-ray. Top arrow indicates the false cord or ventricular band. The lower arrow indicates the vocal cord.

The *laryngograph* is a relatively recent laryngeal investigation for vocal cord movement. Two electrodes are placed on the neck on either side of the larynx from which recordings of the cord vibration are obtained. An oscilloscope displays a wave form and the varying tracings can be related to normal and abnormal voices.

CHAPTER TWO
DISEASES OF THE LARYNX

A doctor when faced with a problem of making a diagnosis is trained to consider the possibilities under the following headings: Congenital; Traumatic; Inflammatory; Neoplastic; Degenerative; and Psychogenic.

Laryngeal diseases which present with voice change will be considered under these headings. The diagnosis of a psychogenic disorder is made after organic disease has been ruled out and this group of disorders is, therefore, always considered last.

CONGENITAL DISORDERS

The larynx is relatively immune to developmental abnormalities. An atresia in which the lumen of the larynx is completely occluded is not compatible with life and is a rare cause of still birth; this gross abnormality is of relevance in that a partial atresia of the larynx may occur. In this disorder, seen in children or adults, there is web joining the vocal cords. A hoarse or abnormally high-pitched voice is associated with a mucosal or fibrous membrane linking the cords across the anterior commissure (Figure 8). The

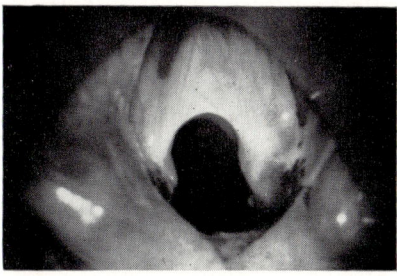

Figure 8 Membrane linking cords across the anterior commissure.

13

appearance of the vocal cords is similar to the adhesion that may form between the vocal cords anteriorly if the cords are 'stripped' surgically to the anterior commissure (see p. 25). If the web is small, the voice change may be minimal and small webs are often not diagnosed until adult life and may be discovered on a routine examination. The anterior commissure is one of the more difficult sites for the ENT surgeon to see on indirect laryngoscopy, so that this lesion may be missed, and the patient diagnosed as a voice production problem with referral for speech therapy. The speech therapist may suspect a congenital web if the response to treatment is unsatisfactory and should discuss the question of further indirect laryngoscopy with the surgeon. If the web is mucous membrane, simple division may suffice as treatment, but frequently there is a thick fibrous link, and division will be followed by an adhesion. It is necessary to secure a plastic splint between the vocal cords anteriorly, while epithelialization occurs and this splint is stitched into the larynx.

Another unusual congenital abnormality of the larynx is *laryngomalacia,* or 'congenital laryngeal stridor'. In this condition, the tissues of the larynx appear to be unusually lax, and the lumen of the larynx is partially occluded by an indrawing of the arytenoids and aryepiglottic folds on inspiration producing an unusual crowing noise. Direct laryngoscopy in these children also shows that there are other abnormalities in the larynx. The epiglottis may be very 'curled', the aryepiglottic folds appear shortened and cord movement is noticed to be lacking in synchrony. There is, however, no apparent difficulty in breathing at rest or on exertion and little or no alteration in the voice. This condition, which is noticed at, or soon after birth, improves gradually and spontaneously, usually well before puberty, without treatment.

TRAUMA TO THE LARYNX

Direct Trauma

Although the larynx is a fairly exposed prominence in the neck, it is protected by the chin; also the mobility of the larynx and flexibility of the cartilages limits damage from external injury. Road traffic accidents are a common cause of crush injury to the larynx and fractures and disruption of the cartilages can occur. Early repair of these injuries is necessary, lest healing and fibrosis occur with laryngeal and tracheal cartilages in poor apposition, so that permanent voice change and airway limitation result. The vocal cords may adhere in the mid-line after a crush injury to the larynx. Tracheostomy is performed in severe direct laryngeal injury as swelling of mucous membrane and disruption of the cartilages will cause airway obstruction.

If repair and reapposition of the larynx and trachea are carried out within several days of laceration and crush injury, there is a good prognosis for both the airway and the voice. The voice and the airway may however be prejudiced if injury to the cricoarytenoid joints limits movement of the cords, or if one or both of the recurrent laryngeal nerves have been severed or irreversibly damaged. If repair of a laryngeal and tracheal injury is delayed and an emergency tracheostomy is the only immediate surgery, a narrowing or stenosis above or below the cords, or at the level of the cords may occur with airway obstruction that means dependence on a tracheostomy. Repair of these injuries is difficult and is not always successful. In cases of tracheal stenosis excision of the stenosed section with end to end anastomoses (the larynx having been mobilized from above and the trachea from below) is often effective. An indwelling stent, small and made of teflon, is often sutured into the larynx and trachea temporarily to maintain a lumen while healing occurs after laryngeal stenosis.

An external blow to the neck may cause internal bruising and swelling of the larynx with little, or no apparent change to the neck externally. Injury to the larynx of this type may occur in sports such as hockey and rugger or result from assault. The hoarseness is often associated with neck pain and stiffness and the patient complains that his voice feels 'tight'; the voice sounds 'tight' and restricted. Indirect laryngoscopy shows bruising and oedema and it is frequently the arytenoid region where the changes are most obvious. Minimal trauma to the neck followed by a marked voice change, in which the laryngeal changes are minimal suggests a functional voice problem triggered off by injury;

such a case can be seen after alleged physical assault. Traumatic lesions settle spontaneously with voice rest.

A direct blow to the neck can also impair the function of the recurrent laryngeal nerves, usually the left which is more vulnerable is affected and hoarseness is due to a cord palsy. This type of recurrent nerve palsy is usually temporary and there is full recovery. The recurrent laryngeal nerves are also at risk from surgical trauma during partial or total thyroidectomy, (see p. 39).

Trauma from Laryngeal Intubation during General Anaesthesia

The vocal cords may be injured at the time of laryngeal intubation for a general anaesthetic. A rubber or plastic tube is placed between the cords and an abrasion to the mucous membrane can be caused by the tube. The usual site for this injury is over the vocal process of the arytenoid cartilage where the mucous membrane is close to the perichondrium; healing in this site is often incomplete and granulation tissue forms where epithelialization of the cords is deficient. The granulation is known as an *intubation granuloma*

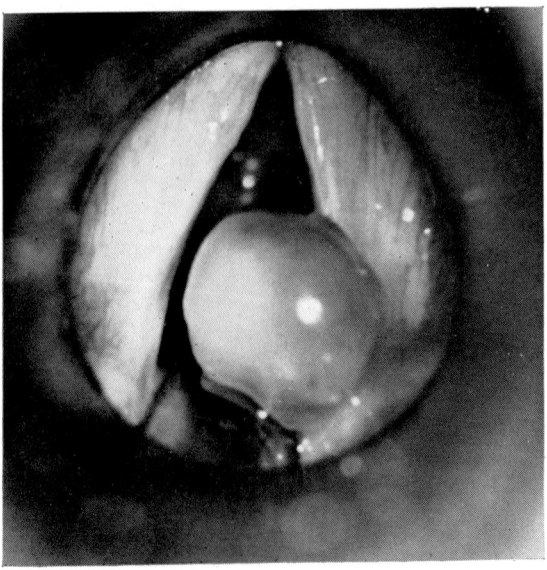

Figure 9 An intubation granuloma.

(Figure 9) and may be a sessile or large pedunculated fibrous swelling. Removal of the granuloma is necessary but due to poor epithelialization over the vocal process the lesion not infrequently recurs necessitating revision operation. It has recently been suggested that zinc sulphate, given orally, reduces the incidence of recurrence of these granulomas and may even cause regression of an established granuloma. The way in which zinc sulphate causes this response is unknown.

The laryngeal tube may also act as an irritant to the laryngeal mucous membrane and hoarseness after intubation may be due to a traumatic laryngitis. A generally reddened mucous membrane is seen on examination and this type of laryngitis may persist for several weeks. Fortunately, good intubation technique has reduced the incidence of granulomas and traumatic laryngitis and these complications are rare.

A more serious danger of laryngeal intubation may develop if too large a tube for the lumen of the trachea is used or if the tube is left in the trachea for a long time. An indwelling laryngeal intubation tube is used on occasions instead of a tracheostomy to ensure the airway and control breathing. If this tube causes undue pressure on the trachea below the cords, pressure ulceration may lead to a narrowing of the lumen and this subglottic laryngeal stenosis may permanently limit the airway and alter the voice.

Trauma from Vocal Abuse

Trauma to the vocal cord can occur as a result of an episode of severe vocal abuse. A person who has indulged in bellowing can produce a haematoma on or near the vocal cord. Examination shows a recent submucosal bleed surrounded by oedema.

Foreign bodies may impact in the larynx and are surprisingly well tolerated, particularly in children. An inhaled fish or meat bone, or a pin, may lodge transversely across the region of the arytenoids and ventricular bands and after the initial sensation of choking and coughing, the cough becomes a relatively minor symptom or may be absent, and hoarseness is the presenting symptom. A laryngeal foreign body should always be considered as a possibility in the diagnosis of a hoarse child.

INFLAMMATIONS OF THE LARYNX

Inflammatory diseases are either acute or chronic.

Acute Laryngitis

Acute laryngitis is a fairly common complication of an upper respiratory tract infection such as a cold. It may develop spontaneously or be precipitated by vocal abuse or heavy smoking at the time of the infection. Professional voice users are particularly vulnerable to acute laryngitis, as the necessity to use their voice not infrequently coincides with an upper respiratory tract infection and the poor voice associated with a cold, which is mainly due to altered nasal resonance tempts the person, if work is continued, to 'force' the voice and precipitate an acute laryngitis. The differential diagnosis of this type of acute laryngitis is a functional aphonia or dysphonia. The patient with a functional voice problem commonly describes the condition as 'laryngitis' and is frequently treated as such by the doctor, for a definite diagnosis cannot be made without indirect laryngoscopy. A functional overlay with acute laryngitis also occurs, and is characterized by a markedly altered voice, with minimal inflammatory changes of the vocal cords on examination.

Examination of the larynx during acute laryngitis shows a bright red laryngeal mucous membrane and in a virulent attack there is pus on the mucosa and pain in the region of the larynx, associated with the hoarseness. The treatment for acute laryngitis is with antibiotics, inhalations and voice rest. A mild attack will settle with voice rest, but patients who persist with excessive talking and smoking during an attack of laryngitis may develop persistent hoarseness due to chronic laryngitis. Lozenges and laryngeal sprays have little place in the treatment of acute laryngitis, but a singer or speaker who is compelled to use his voice may be helped for a short time with a laryngeal spray containing an antihistamine or vasoconstrictor, which reduces the swelling of the mucous membrane and the excess mucus production.

Chronic Laryngitis

Chronic laryngitis is characterized by persistent hoarseness varying in severity. It may develop from an acute laryngitis (in which a period of voice rest has been ignored) or it may develop gradually as a result of prolonged laryngeal irritation or infection. Irritants that cause changes in the mucous membrane of the larynx are often environmental and related to the patient's occupation; a dusty or dirty atmosphere such as that containing tar or chemical fumes can set up a persistent irritative laryngitis. Speaking, and shouting orders may coincide with heavy manual work. The ventricular bands and vocal cords are adducted during lifting of heavy objects and simultaneous use of the voice such as shouting orders is a factor in chronic laryngitis. Smoking may, in some patients, cause little obvious change in the upper respiratory tract, whereas in others the entire mucous membrane is reddened, although heavy smoking is invariably associated with some degree of change in the laryngeal mucous membrane. Excessive use of the voice and faulty voice production also cause chronic inflammatory changes. Frequently, all these factors contribute to a persistently hoarse voice; a man undertaking heavy manual work in a dusty and noisy atmosphere may smoke heavily, bellow at his colleagues, and at weekends give excessive vocal support at a football match. Alcohol may also be a factor in perpetuating hoarseness; alcohol causes dilation of the vessels of the mucous membrane and in excess may act as an irritant to the pharynx and larynx.

The changes seen in the larynx in chronic laryngitis vary. In men, there is usually a dull, red mucous membrane with a thickening of the ventricular bands. This thickening may be marked and in some cases the ventricular bands meet in the mid-line on phonation and are being used to produce the hoarse voice. In severe, chronic laryngitis, white patches, or leukoplakia may develop on the thickened mucous membrane. Leukoplakia is commonest on the vocal cords but also occurs on the ventricular bands and on the arytenoids. Microscopic examination shows that the white area is due to a keratinized or horny epithelium and this condition is known as *hyperkeratosis*. Hyperkeratosis is a premalignant condition increasing the likelihood of laryngeal cancer. It may also be a reversible condition if the irritant factors to the larynx are removed.

In women, there tends to be a different clinical type of chronic laryngitis. The commonest cause is vocal abuse and faulty voice production. The personality is often that of a rather tense woman with a nervous cough, who may smoke and tends to talk excessively and loudly. Someone involved in shouting at a deaf person with whom they live may develop laryngitis, as may a mother who shrieks at her children. People involved in frequent and long telephone conversations may alter their voice production when using the telephone, tending to force their voice or shout. The commonest change in the larynx is an oedema of the vocal cords so that the free border, instead of being firm and white, is lax, grey and polypoid; a large polyp may develop on the margin of the cord. Oedema tends to be a more conspicuous and common finding than the hyperaemia and hypertrophy seen in the male larynx.

It may not be practical to treat hoarseness due to chronic laryngitis. An environment and occupation that cannot be changed, or a person who persists in smoking, prevent effective treatment. The changes, however, of chronic laryngitis are frequently reversible; cutting out tobacco may result in the disappearance of long-standing changes in the mucous membrane and leukoplakia may regress. Vocal cords with oedematous margins may return to normal with advice and help in establishing correct voice production, and enlarged ventricular bands may also similarly improve. Vocal cord polypi, however, require surgical removal and will not respond to conservative treatment.

Vocal cord nodules   Vocal cord nodules are a special type of localized chronic laryngitis. These lesions tend to occur in those who use their voice professionally and are therefore called 'singer's nodules' (Figure 10). They may also occur in tense and excitable personalities who tend to chatter excessively. A housewife harassed by children and shouting instructions is a candidate for vocal cord nodule formation; this personality may find organization of the children and

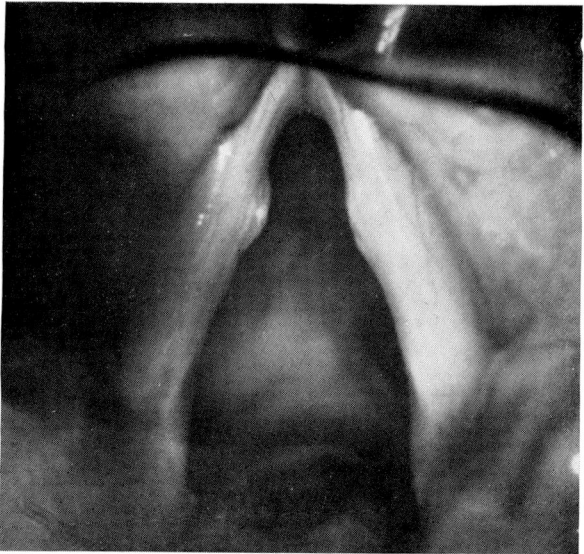

Figure 10   Vocal cord nodules ('Singer's' nodules).

household difficult, and may live in some disorganization. The discipline that speech therapy for vocal cord nodules involves may, therefore, be difficult for this type of patient to acquire. Although singer's nodules are a hazard of the professional voice user, the type of patient susceptible to the generalized type of chronic laryngitis that has been described, may also develop nodules. Nodules may be associated with a generalized laryngitis, but usually occur in an otherwise normal, or near-normal larynx.

The voice has a characteristic hoarseness, not always unattractive, which is used by some actresses who may wish to perpetuate their vocal nodules. In many cases, however, nodules are not compatible with a socially acceptable voice and a person singing professionally is severely limited with nodules and will probably be unable to work. Those with good voice training rarely develop nodules, unless their vocal commitment is too heavy. Nodules are found in those called upon to talk or sing to excess with little or no training in voice production. Singing against considerable background noise, with inadequate amplification, and fulfilling too many singing commitments are all additional factors predisposing to vocal nodules. Attention to singing technique and limiting singing commitments are necessary, in addition to speech therapy.

The earliest change seen in the larynx of a patient who is a candidate for nodule formation is an oedema which develops between the anterior third and posterior two-thirds of the free margins of the vocal cords. The oedema at this site will settle with voice rest, but if ignored a thickening of the cord margin develops. Firm nodules form which are usually bilateral although not always symmetrical. The site on the vocal cord is constant.

Vocal cord nodules are not an uncommon cause of hoarseness in children and they may occur for a variety of reasons. A child from a large family where competitive shouting is necessary for attention may develop extremely large nodules from the age of four upwards. These are sometimes known as 'screamer's' nodes, which is an apt description. A constant background noise from domestic machinery such as dishwashers, food mixers or polishers may contribute to the establishment of vocal cord nodules for the child who is constantly raising the voice in order to be heard. The persistent use of the record player or transistor radio by another member of the family also adds to background noise. One also has to remember that the background noise level in the average school may be considerable. 'Screamer's' nodules tend to occur in boys who are sports fans, supporting or playing in school teams and belonging to clubs and organizations, all of which may demand considerable vocal support.

Contact ulcers Contact ulcers are another variant of chronic laryngitis resulting from a chronic misuse of the voice. This is a superficial ulceration of the vocal cord mucosa in the region of the vocal process. This ulceration is more common in males who have tried to lower the pitch of their voice or have tried to increase volume by incorrect methods such as forcing air from the neck region; the voice sounds, in fact, as if it is being 'forced' through the larynx.

Treatment of vocal cord nodules Although a small nodule may regress with voice rest and subsequent voice training, larger, or established thickening of the vocal cord will require removal. Removal of the nodule alone, however, will not restore a normal voice and the nodule will recur if the underlying faulty voice production is not corrected. It is, therefore, necessary for the voice of a patient with singer's nodules to be assessed and treated preoperatively by the speech therapist and for the patient to attend speech therapy postoperatively. There are, however, no serious complications of nodules and if the patient prefers the hoarseness to treatment and if treatment is impractical, as it may be in the case of a mother with several children, no harm will come if the nodules are ignored.

There needs to be close cooperation between the ENT surgeon and speech therapist when treating vocal cord nodules. The type of person with nodules often has too many duties and obligations, and tends to want quick results. They are not willing to be on a strict regime of limited voice use and good voice production. The idea of an operation, where the work and effort involved is carried out by the surgeon, appeals to the patient rather more than having to attend for speech therapy. The patient may well, therefore, press for surgical removal of the nodules and the reason why surgery is not in itself curative must be made clear. It is important to explain that the hoarseness is primarily the result of faulty voice production and this has caused the nodule formation. It is the voice production, as well as the nodules, that cause the hoarseness and simple removal of the nodules does not result in a return of normal voice.

If the surgeon advises speech therapy prior to surgery, the length of treatment should be discussed (*e.g.* speech therapy for two months with review at one month). The nodules may enlarge if the patient does not adhere to the voice regime prescribed by the speech therapist, but if the patient is using the voice better there may be a regression of the nodules.

If the nodules are well established and it is felt they are unlikely to diminish with speech therapy and the decision is taken to operate, the speech therapist's task is lessened if treatment is begun prior to surgery. It is often easier to gain the patient's cooperation at this stage if posture work and breathing can be started and some progress can be shown. The patient is then more likely to continue to cooperate after surgery. The speech therapist can play an active part after the operation in emphasizing the need for voice rest which most surgeons recommend. Work on resonance and the production of an easy note can be started about ten days after surgery.

Speech therapists vary in their opinion about the value of relaxation in treatment. Relaxation, however, has a very important part to play in the treatment of vocal cord nodules. The patient must be helped to become aware of the need to relax, 'ease down' and so slow down and take life at a more leisurely pace. Supine relaxation as part of the treatment may be needed and general discussions on relaxation are helpful. Voice exercises help patients to feel more relaxed and at ease; this probably stems from the relaxed atmosphere of a speech therapy department and as they repeat the exercises at home, they try to achieve the same feeling. Posture work may need more attention when treating singer's nodules than with any other voice disorder. Correct breathing will more easily be achieved if the patient is easy and relaxed. The characteristic speaking voice faults in those with nodules are poor breathing, rapid speech and limited nasal resonance.

With the screamer's nodules of children, it is necessary to limit or stop their vocal support at games and not to allow it to be resumed until there is progress and improvement in the voice. The school's cooperation should be sought; the child should be excused singing classes and he should be stopped from shouting. This is difficult to control in the playground but it may, in some cases, be possible to lessen the time spent in the playground if the child can go home for lunch and not return to school until the beginning of the afternoon session. The regime must be firm, but the praise lavish for every success as well as a reward being made: this can well be some easing of the voice restriction regime. It is helpful if the mother attends to have her 'sit in' on the treatment session. She can hear and see what is required for good voice production and can, therefore, help the child more easily. The mother can be asked to produce correct sounds and the patient can correct her if necessary.

Treatment of contact ulcers   Contact ulcers are treated by the speech therapist first by making the patient, usually a man, aware of the natural pitch of his voice, which he has unconsciously altered. Correct voice production technique and correct ways of increasing volume are targets. Persistent, unnecessary 'throat clearing' is characteristic in a patient with contact ulcers and this habit can be discouraged.

NEOPLASMS OF THE LARYNX

A neoplasm is a new growth; it is either benign or malignant. Benign tumours are characteristically local swellings which may increase greatly in size and compress adjacent structures. A malignant growth usually invades and destroys the structure involved and those adjacent to it; it also spreads via the lymphatics to the lymph nodes, and may spread via the blood stream to further sites in the body. Cancers are malignant tumours of which the commonest type in the larynx is the carcinoma. Spread of cancer to lymph nodes and elsewhere via the blood stream is known as metastasis. Benign tumours do not metastasize.

Benign Lesions

Polyps are common benign lesions, presenting with hoarseness. A polyp may form on a vocal cord with oedema resulting from chronic laryngitis, or it may arise spontaneously in an otherwise normal larynx. Large polyps tend to be pedunculated so that they move above and below the vocal cords on inspiration and expiration (Figure 11). It is possible for a large polyp to be missed on examination by indirect laryngoscopy when it has fallen below the cord on inspiration and remained in this position. A patient with a vocal cord polyp tends to develop an altered voice production in an attempt to produce a normal voice, so that surgical removal of the polyp does not necessarily result in an immediate cure of the hoarseness. Postoperative speech therapy is usually effective in restoring the voice. Polyps involving both vocal cords and extending to the anterior commissure present a surgical problem; if both cords are 'stripped' anteriorly, an adhesion, or web may form at the commissure. With polyps of both cords the polyp is removed to the

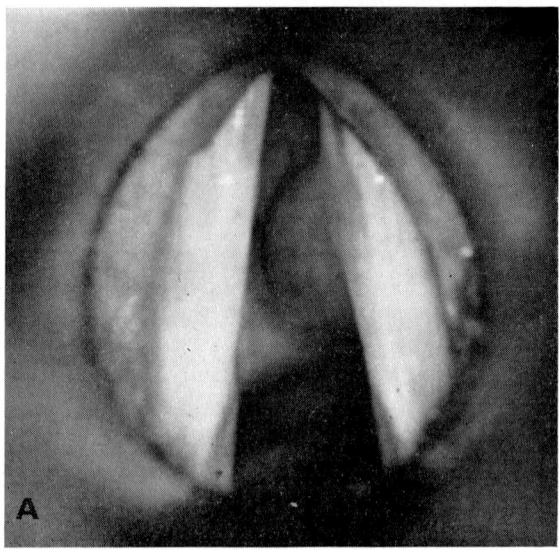

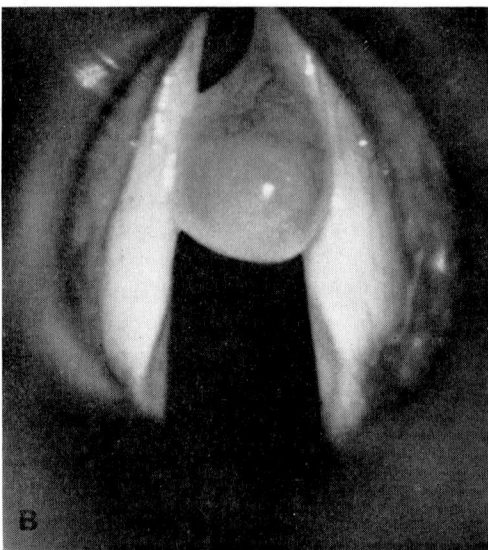

Figure 11 A large vocal cord polyp. A, the polyp is drawn below the vocal cord on inspiration and is not obvious an examination. B, the polyp becomes obvious on expiration when blown upwards onto the surface of the cord.

anterior commissure on one cord only and the mucosa of the anterior third of the other cord is left intact. Subsequently when the larynx has re-epithelialized, the remaining polyp can be removed. A laryngeal web resulting from surgery is difficult to treat and a recurrence of the adhesion usually follows simple division to the anterior commissure. It is necessary, therefore, to secure a plastic splint between the cords anteriorly until the cords have epithelialized.

Firm fibrous tumours also occur in the larynx called fibromas and excision by direct laryngoscopy is usually curative. Papillomas are important benign tumours of the larynx. These wart-like swellings with an irregular surface may occur as a solitary lesion in an adult and have a tendency to recur following removal, so that follow-up and periodic direct laryngoscopy may be necessary. More commonly, however, papilloma occur in children and are extensive and multiple and known as *juvenile papilloma of the larynx*. These lesions must be excluded in a child presenting with hoarseness; if ignored, the papillomas become extensive and occlude the laryngeal inlet causing inspiratory obstruction and maybe total obstruction of the airway. Eighty percent of juvenile papillomas occur in the first five years of life; the onset may be in infancy and a baby with a persistently hoarse cry should be suspected of having papillomas. The breathing, if the papillomas are extensive, is noisy and difficulty on inspiration is known as stridor. This is different from the difficulty in breathing in asthma where the problem is on expiration due to spasm of the muscles surrounding the bronchioles (bronchospasm).

The treatment of juvenile papillomas is not easy as recurrence follows removal. Periodic microlaryngoscopy and removal is necessary to ensure that a clear airway is maintained. As with removal of vocal cord polyps, care must be taken not to remove papillomas from both cords anteriorly at the same operation. The risk of a permanent fibrous scar webbing the anterior commissure, which accentuates the hoarseness and further reduces the airway, is very real. Severe airway obstruction may necessitate a tracheostomy; this operation is to be avoided if possible for the papillomas tend to 'seed' and form in the trachea at the site of the tracheostomy opening.

If it does become necessary to perform a tracheostomy, it is extremely important for the child to be fitted with a tube with a speaking valve, this ensures that while air on inspiration is taken through the tracheostome, air on expiration is directed through the larynx: the valve at the opening of the tracheostomy tube hinges inwards on inspiration, opening the tube, and closes on expiration due to the pressure of expired air. It is now well recognized that the larynx of children with tracheostomies who do not use a speaking valve does not develop normally and remains small. Mucus also is not expelled from the larynx if air is not directed up through the cords on expiration and this prejudices normal laryngeal physiology and growth.

The cause of juvenile papillomas is unknown but fortunately they tend to regress at puberty and it is uncommon for them to persist to adult life. They remain benign lesions and do not develop into carcinoma. Treatment, other than meticulous removal which may be combined with diathermy to the base of the papilloma, is experimental although there is evidence that ultrasound therapy may be effective. It is extremely rare for a child with papillomas to achieve a normal voice despite meticulous surgical removal, and speech therapy helps these children to avoid developing faulty or forced voice production. It is also helpful for the speech therapist to see the child and assess the voice before surgery to remove papillomas. There is not infrequently a superimposed psychogenic voice problem for the child may be unsettled by the mother's obvious concern about the abnormal voice and by other people's response to the voice. Also, repeated visits to hospital over many years for removal of the papillomas is another disturbing factor for the child and parents. The main aim in speech therapy work with these children is for controlled breathing. Little, if any, direct work can of course be achieved with the very young child. Breathing can be guided by the therapist's hand whilst sitting the child on the therapist's knee. Since these children are frequently tense and anxious, relaxation games can be helpful. The speech therapist should also be alert to detect a functional component in the problem voice.

It is necessary to exclude laryngeal papillomas in every case of a *persistently hoarse child*, but laryngeal nodules are probably the commonest lesion causing hoarseness and foreign bodies also occur. A functional dysphonia is also not uncommon in children and is a further diagnosis to be considered.

Cysts form when a mucus-secreting gland is either obstructed or ruptured so that mucus is released into the surrounding tissues. A swelling usually in the supraglottic region is the commonest cyst in the larynx but cysts may also be concealed below the cords and may not be easily detected particularly in the small larynx of a child. These are not tumours but are a benign laryngeal swelling.

Malignant Lesions

The squamous cell carcinoma involving the vocal cord is the most common laryngeal cancer. Persistent hoarseness is the presenting symptom, and examination of the larynx shows an irregular ulcer of the vocal cord (Figure 12). Pain is

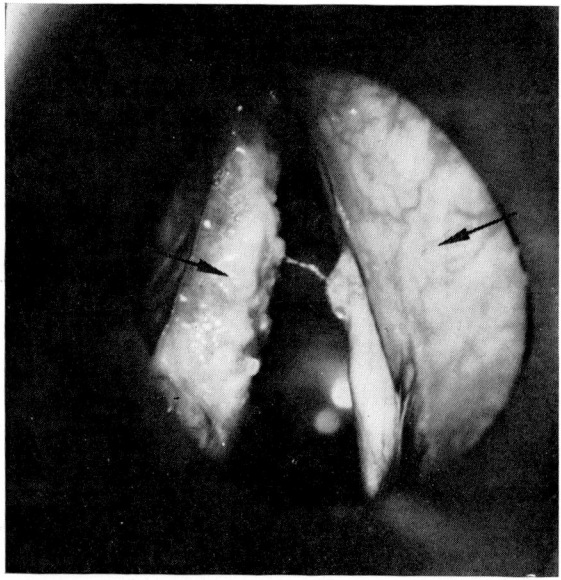

Figure 12   Carcinoma of the vocal cord.

uncommon with early cancer of the larynx and any symptom other than hoarseness suggests a more advanced lesion.

Almost all carcinomas of the vocal cord occur in those who smoke and a carcinoma may develop in a long-standing chronic laryngitis in which there is hyperkeratosis. An early cord carcinoma has an excellent chance of complete cure with radiotherapy. There are a number of reasons for this good prognosis; a small lesion of the cord will cause hoarseness so that the tumour presents early; a persistent hoarseness is now well recognized by patients and doctors as a significant symptom requiring examination of the larynx. The vocal cord is pale due to relatively few blood vessels, and it also has few lymphatics; hence, spread of the tumour via the lymphatics to the lymph nodes or via the bloodstream is very uncommon in an early lesion. The vocal cords although enclosed within the thyroid cartilage are placed fairly close to the surface of the skin and the deep X-rays can be directed with great accuracy on to the carcinoma with little involvement of the surrounding tissues and little scatter. A normal voice and larynx follows radiotherapy in about 80 to 90% of cases of cord carcinomas. A dry mouth due to damage to the mucous glands occurs but this symptom settles. The dose of radiotherapy given is about 5000 rads in daily doses over six weeks. Nausea during the treatment is a troublesome side effect and this is controlled with tablets such as Stemetil (prochlorperazine). Many patients will continue their job while attending for their course of radiotherapy. The treatment involves only several minutes daily under radiotherapy.

Voice problems may occur in those who are involved in a job requiring excess use of the voice and work in an irritant atmosphere. An irritative laryngitis may develop unnecessarily if these factors are ignored. Patients undergoing radiotherapy for carcinoma of the larynx should be forbidden to smoke and cigarette smoking after radiotherapy predisposes to recurrence.

Before the development of modern radiotherapy, the laryngofissure operation was the treatment for early vocal cord carcinoma. Good results were obtained, similar to those achieved with radiotherapy, with excision of the vocal cord. With radiotherapy, however, a normal voice is achieved whereas a laryngofissure is always followed by persistent hoarseness. This operation still has a place on the rare occasions when a small vocal cord tumour persists after radiotherapy; laryngofissure may also be necessary for cord carcinoma in countries where radiotherapy is not available. Only if a cord carcinoma fails to respond to radiotherapy and extends beyond the vocal process, is the operation of laryngectomy necessary.

Carcinoma of the larynx may develop above the vocal cord in the region of the ventricular band and is called a *supraglottic carcinoma*, or the lesion may be on the under surface of the vocal cord and upper trachea, *subglottic carcinoma*. The lesions on the vocal cord are called *glottic carcinoma*, and about 70% of the lesions are glottic, 20% supraglottic and 10% subglottic.

The supra- and subglottic carcinomas have a considerably worse prognosis than glottic lesions. The hoarseness may not occur until the lesion enlarges to involve the vocal cord and the supra- and subglottic regions are more vascular with more lymphatics which predisposes to local and general (systemic) spread of disease. The initial treatment is with radiotherapy, but laryngectomy is more frequently required after treatment, for these lesions do not respond as well as glottic carcinoma. A voice that remains hoarse after radiotherapy suggests residual carcinoma. A poor voice with an abnormal laryngeal appearance on indirect laryngoscopy such as persistent swelling of the arytenoids, necessitates direct laryngoscopy and biopsy. If the histological examination proves carcinoma still to be present, surgery, usually a total laryngectomy, is necessary. Operation is usually carried out six to eight weeks after completion of radiotherapy; the neck tissues are more vascular soon after radiotherapy and postoperative healing may be poor. Eight weeks following radiotherapy the neck tissues slowly become firm and fibrotic and surgical dissection is more difficult; the eight-week time after radiotherapy is, therefore, the best time for surgery.

Carcinoma of the pyriform fossa involves the lateral wall of the larynx. Pain and difficulty in swallowing occur with the pyriform fossa lesions associated with hoarseness when the larynx is involved. It is not uncommon for pain from laryngeal or pyriform fossa carcinomas to be referred to the ear. The vagus nerve which supplies the larynx also has a branch supplying the ear drum and external auditory meatus. The phenomenon of pain being felt in a site not directly involved with disease, but having the same nerve supply, is not uncommon and is known as referred pain. Disease in the lower molar teeth or tonsils may also cause earache and are other examples of referred pain.

DEGENERATIVE CONDITIONS OF THE LARYNX

Tissues tend to become more lax with age as the elasticity becomes less; this change is particularly apparent in the skin The voice varies less in tone and pitch in old age and may sound monotonous. A tremulous voice may also develop. The voice in old age is also less strong and this is usually accepted unless the patient is a singer and complains of loss of range of voice. Examination shows some bowing of the vocal cords and this is a natural ageing process and is not amenable to treatment. Some air will, therefore, escape on adduction and account for the loss of power.

The joints of the larynx, particularly the cricoarytenoid joints are not infrequently involved in rheumatoid arthritis. Impairment of mobility of the cord and fixation of the cords into a near mid-line position may occur. In severe rheumatoid involvement, however, the cords become fixed so near the mid-line that airway obstruction occurs and the patient presents with shortness of breath on exertion and stridor.

PSYCHOGENIC VOICE DISORDERS

There are three psychogenic voice disorders; functional aphonia, functional dysphonia and mutism. Puberphonia may also be considered as a type of dysphonia, although the unbroken voice may be a hormonal disorder and not always psychosomatic.

Functional Aphonia

Functional aphonia is the commonest psychogenic voice disorder. The voice loss presents with a classical, hardly audible, 'mouthed' whisper. Women are more frequently affected than men and are usually in the younger age group or at the menopause. It is a manifestation of a relatively superficial psychiatric disorder and tends to follow an emotional upset. Although a single emotional crisis may cause functional aphonia, it is more frequently due to a number of relatively minor problems having a cumulative effect. The patient may, therefore, not be aware of any single factor or worry and may deny any emotional problem when the history is first taken. It is unusual for the patients to require treatment from a psychiatrist and normal voice is rapidly achieved with speech therapy. There is a tendency for this condition to recur in some people at times of emotional stress. This type of voice is also frequently labelled 'a laryngitis' and may be treated as such, if the characteristics of functional aphonia are not recognized.

Examination of the larynx shows normal anatomy, but the movement of the cords is abnormal; there is inability to adduct normally on attempted phonation. If the patient is asked to cough the cords do adduct fully, but rapidly abduct. This condition, therefore, is not simply a failure of adduction but a failure to *maintain adduction* on phonation.

If possible the speech therapist should see these patients without delay after the ENT consultation, for the voice is regained more easily and quickly the shorter the period of aphonia. The patient may be somewhat distressed by his first vist to a hospital outpatient department, and the indirect laryngoscopy, which is uncomfortable, may have further unsettled the patient. The relief, however, in being reassured that there is no sign of serious disease should not be underestimated and in their relief they will often talk more freely. If there is a delay between the initial visit to the doctor and the first speech therapy appointment, the patient may start to realize that worry and distress may have a part in the voice loss and some patients will build up a resistance to speech therapy.

The skill in handling the patient with functional aphonia

is to extract the necessary information at the interview and so to be aware of all the possible causes. The return of voice often comes when the patients begin to discuss their problems and they relax and may cry, so the beginnings of voice can be heard and this can then be pursued. It is also helpful to give some basic voice exercises; this will ensure that the voice is used easily and that the regained voice is maintained. Further visits are often then more acceptable to the patient. The speech therapist has further opportunities to verify that all the patient's problems have come to light and been discussed. One frequently helps by applying plain commonsense.

If the speech therapist suspects that there are deep-seated underlying problems unlikely to respond to speech therapy the patient should be referred back to the ENT surgeon, as referral for a psychiatric opinion may be necessary. During speech therapy the overall management responsibility for the patient is maintained by the referring ENT surgeon.

It is helpful when a child or adolescent is accompanied by a parent, for the interview to take place in two parts; first the parent is interviewed, then the patient. Some young patients are not willing to discuss their home problems with their parents present, but in the clinic situation, with the help of the speech therapist, they will feel more able to talk. Often the problems are of a minor nature but nevertheless distressing to the child or adolescent. Frequently as in the adult it is an accumulation of a number of small things. The parent may suspect that the speech therapist is looking for a deep-seated problem and they need to be assured that it is an accumulation of minor worries that are more likely to have given rise to the voice loss. The school can sometimes give help with information about school progress and the child's ability to get on with the other children.

In those cases where voice is not regained when discussing problems, other methods must be used such as sighing out a sound 'ah' on the outgoing breath, or a hum; attention should be drawn away from the neck. The hum can be felt by putting the finger on the nose, or the idea of directing the voice well ahead can be employed.

Functional Dysphonia

The voice of a functional dysphonic may sound like one with a genuine laryngeal lesion for there is either a marked hoarseness or a curious alteration in the voice. The diagnosis of a psychogenic disturbance is confirmed when examination shows a normal larynx. Functional dysphonias are not uncommon in children with emotional problems and a full, careful history usually makes clear the factors that underlie the faulty voice production. They respond well, like the functional aphonias, to speech therapy and psychiatric help is rarely required.

The key to speech therapy treatment is a full case history so that all possible stresses in this condition can be detected. In many cases the voice begins to alter as the patients talk about their problems. Many people are in need of an impartial, but sympathetic listener; the general practitioner may not have sufficient time during surgery hours to listen, nor is it always easy for the patient to talk freely in an outpatient department. There are often too many people about, and interruptions to the consultation may occur. Sometimes the problems are insoluble, but in discussion the patient may be given another view and so be able to accept or come to terms with a difficulty. Occasionally, the main worry may not be discussed at the interview, although the therapist may be aware that a certain area is not being discussed as fully as others and it is only later when the patient has regained a normal voice that the main underlying concern is discussed. As with the cases of functional aphonia the emotional factors are often not deep-seated. Sometimes, normal voice begins to return during the history-taking. This voice is then encouraged and may become normal, or near-normal as the tensions are released.

When there is no sign of normal voice throughout the case history, other methods are used. Most of these patients are overconscious of the neck and the region of the larynx and it is useful to divert attention away from these areas by concentration on good posture with exercises to relax shoulders and neck. Then progress is made and good, easy breathing, working through several exercises controlling outgoing air. The patient can then be asked to sigh out the air in a prolonged 'aaah' and when this is achieved, to hum the air out, feeling it by the nose. Relaxation is encouraged to prevent forcing and effort to produce normal voice. When the hum is obtained easily, this is followed by a vowel sound and then a hum followed by a word so that voice is being used almost before the patient is aware of it. The use of voice exercises not only allows the therapist to verify that the voice is continuing to improve but gives further opportunities of discussion at later appointments.

Mutism

Mutism is mentioned to complete the types of psychogenic voice disorders but the condition is seen by psychiatrists and rarely seen by speech therapists and ENT surgeons. In most cases, the development of complete absence of voice with previous normal speech is due to malingering. Cases have been described in which the voice has been absent for many years following an accident, during which time medicolegal procedings are taking place. After settlement of the case, the voice has returned. The case has also been described of a person committed to prison who did not speak for several years but spoke normally on release.

Mutism may also occur intermittently and such episodes are commonly due to hysteria. Children as young as three and four may also produce similar bouts of elective mutism in which speech, hitherto normal, is absent. Although mutism is therefore usually psychogenic, speech disturbances varying from aphonia to mutism may be caused by an idiosyncrasy to the phenothiazine group of drugs (this includes the tranquillizer drugs), even when given in average doses. Questions are met either with total silence or a whisper is received in response to repeated questioning. More rarely, frontal lobe brain tumours may disturb speech and cause mutism.

Puberphonia

Puberphonia is the persistence of the unbroken male voice. Although this condition may be due to hormone imbalance or a psychiatric problem, most cases are due to faulty voice production which may be related to a superficial emotional problem, and respond well to speech therapy. It is important that the questions of hormone imbalance or psychiatric disturbance have been investigated before the patient is referred for speech therapy.

Overuse and misuse of the voice while it is breaking is one cause of puberphonia. A boy may, for example, be due to sing a part and has been persuaded to continue although the voice is just beginning to change. The young will tend to conform and the boy with an early voice break may well be so embarrassed by his deep voice that he will try and force to obtain a higher tone which he may not be able to alter later on.

The aim in treating puberphonia is to obtain a low note and see that this is maintained. The first part is comparatively easy, the second part less so. The case history is taken with further questions regarding any voice break and details of shaving. Enquiries should be made to establish whether the patient has girl friends; the male homosexual who takes the female role in a partnership may well have a high pitched voice which he may not wish to alter.

It is useful to record the patient's voice in general conversation. This can be played back immediately so that he is fully aware of the sound of his voice. As many of these patients are overconscious of the neck and larynx region, it is helpful to draw attention away from these areas. It is effective to ask the patient to hum or speak while feeling the vibration of the sound by placing his finger on the dorsion of his nose. It may be more helpful to begin to obtain the low voice before giving an explanation of voice production. Good posture is established and then breathing work should be started with considerable emphasis on breathing out. The low note can sometimes be obtained by making the patient produce a humming noise and feel the nose. If this fails, then a cough or glottal noises can be used. The therapist should proceed to humming, vowel sounds, and finally aim at the production of words.

Frequently, the boy will be concerned that the deep voice is peculiar and it is helpful in persuading acceptance of the deep voice to make a recording and compare it to the original voice, playing both back to the patient.

MISCELLANEOUS VOICE DISORDERS

Recurrent Laryngeal Nerve Palsy

The recurrent laryngeal branch of the vagus nerve (Xth cranial nerve) supplies the muscles which move the vocal cords and it also supplies sensation to the mucous membrane of the trachea up to the vocal cords. The left recurrent laryngeal nerve has a longer course than the right; it descends into the thorax and winds round the aorta to ascend in the groove between the oesophagus and trachea before entering the larynx. The left recurrent laryngeal nerve is closely related to the ligamentum arteriosum, linking the arch of the aorta to the pulmonary vein, and also it is related to the lymph nodes at the hilum of the lung. The lobes of the thyroid gland are adjacent to the recurrent laryngeal nerves, as are the paratracheal lymph nodes, in the groove between the oesophagus and trachea.

Loss of function of one recurrent laryngeal nerve causes immobility of the cord on that side. Because of failure to totally adduct the cords, the voice is hoarse, and it has a characteristic 'breathy' quality with audible escape of air on phonation; the volume is poor and can only partly be increased with effort. The voice tends to be monotonous with few changes in pitch. The laugh, too, is altered and the patient's companions may comment on its peculiar new quality. There is also a loss of power of expulsion of the cough; this is normally not a handicap, but when associated with chest lesions such as chronic bronchitis, this presents a problem of inability to satisfactorily clear the excess sputum.

Examination of the larynx shows the immobile cord in a position just lateral to the mid-line and at a slightly lower level than the normal vocal cord for the arytenoid falls slightly anteriorly when paralysed. On phonation, the mobile cord adducts but there is a failure of complete apposition to the immobile cord and air escapes.

Causes   Trauma to the recurrent laryngeal nerves in the chest or neck may cause a temporary or permanent loss of function. An external blow to the side of the neck may cause a temporary cord palsy on that side. In the operation of partial or total thyroidectomy, although great care is taken to preserve the recurrent laryngeal nerves, one or both may occasionally be damaged. If there is complete division of the nerve, the palsy will persist; the nerve may be involved in bruising or swelling of the tissues and when the haematoma has resolved, and oedema settled, function returns. The recurrent laryngeal nerves are at greater risk in revision thyroid surgery when scarring from the previous operation may have altered the anatomy and course of the nerve and the nerve may, furthermore, be more difficult for the surgeon to locate when obscured in scar tissue. Before thyroid surgery, the vocal cord movement is examined by an ENT surgeon to confirm that there is no preoperative nerve palsy. A thyroid cancer may damage the nerve and pressure from a benign thyroid swelling may also impair the nerve's function.

Injury to the thoracic portion of the left recurrent laryngeal nerve may follow thoracotomy for ligation of a congenitally patent ductus arteriosus for the nerve winds round the ductus before ascending into the neck.

Metastases in the hilar or cervical lymph nodes adjacent to the oesophagus will also cause a cord palsy if the recurrent laryngeal nerve is involved. Lung carcinoma with secondary involvement of the hilar lymph nodes is now one of the commonest causes of left cord palsy. These cases occur with relatively advanced lung cancer with a poor prognosis and radiotherapy, rather than lung resection, is the treatment.

Pressure on the left nerve may also come from the left atrium of the heart when this is enlarged due to heart failure from a narrow mitral valve (mitral stenosis). A distension of the arch of the aorta due to a weakness in the arterial wall (syphilitic aneurism) was, in the past, a common cause of pressure and loss of movement of the left cord, but since penicillin has been available to treat syphilis, this cause of cord palsy is a relative rarity.

A patient presenting with hoarseness due to a cord palsy requires, therefore, thorough investigation for diagnosis and a chest X-ray is essential. Despite the many known lesions damaging the recurrent laryngeal nerves, in about one third of cases presenting with cord palsy, no cause is found and these are described as idiopathic. It is usually the left cord that is affected but the right cord may also be involved. Both cords are not affected at the same time.

Idiopathic cord palsies present with the characteristic hoarseness. In many cases, spontaneous recovery of cord movement occurs within nine months or a year. Although treatment does not influence return of cord movement, it is important for a patient with a cord palsy to have speech therapy. A patient with one immobile cord can, with attempts to produce a normal voice, develop a laryngitis and an increase in hoarseness. Speech therapy enables the patient to produce the most satisfactory voice that can be produced with movement of one vocal cord and may actually assist in early compensatory adduction by the mobile cord.

If recovery of cord movement has not occurred within a year, it is almost certain that the paralysis is permanent. Not infrequently, the mobile cord compensates or 'overcloses' to produce complete or near-complete adduction. If compensation is full, a normal voice is achieved and some patients, even with a permanent cord palsy therefore have a satisfactory voice. In most cases, however, of a persisting cord palsy the voice remains inadequate. The condition can be treated with a teflon injection lateral to the vocal cord (p. 57–58). This serves to increase the bulk of the immobile cord so that it reaches the mid-line and the normal cord can then adduct without air escape on phonation.

If both recurrent laryngeal nerves are damaged, the cords take up a position near the mid-line and the problem is one of airway obstruction rather than voice disturbance. Severe limitation of breathing on inspiration occurs, and is accentuated by any exertion; a tracheostomy is often necessary as an emergency. This type of situation may occur when both cords are damaged during a thyroidectomy but fortunately this is a rare complication.

Treatment The speech therapist will help the patient to use the altered voice mechanism to the best advantage. Encouragement to get maximum mobility from the mobile cord is achieved by glottal and pushing exercises. The glottal stop sound is requested or a firm, short cough and these are combined with vowel sounds. The patient may be asked to push against a piece of furniture and then emit the characteristic grunt involved in such an effort. On heavy lifting the vocal cords are fully adducted at the moment the muscles of the thorax, neck and arms are involved in the maximum effort. This tendency of the cords to adduct is therefore encouraged by this exercise. Advice is given to remember to breathe in more frequently while speaking and so compensate for the air waste. There is instruction to learn to recognize the difference between the sound of voice with an adequate air supply and the reverse of this.

Myxoedema

When the thyroid gland is underactive (hypothyroidism) there is often a thickening of the submucosal tissue of the larynx causing hoarseness. The appearance of the larynx in myxoedema resembles a chronic laryngitis.

Androgenic Hoarseness

It is important in history-taking to ask every patient what tablets they are taking. A patient who has made a routine of taking a certain tablet for years may overlook to mention this unless specifically asked. Many tablets have side effects which may be relevant to the presenting symptom. Some tranquillizers for example, cause dryness of the mouth, the contraceptive pill may give rise to headaches, and aspirin if taken to excess causes a ringing noise in the ears (tinnitus). Hormone tablets used to control heavy or irregular periods, or similar tablets used at the menopause, may contain oestrogens combined with a small dose of androgen (the male sex hormone). If such tablets are taken for a long time, the first side effect is in the larynx and a subtle alteration in the voice, particularly noticed in those who sing, precedes a deeper and more hoarse voice with other signs of virilization. This voice change, if detected and diagnosed early, may be reversible, but when a deeper voice is established it tends to persist after the hormone tablet is stopped.

CHAPTER THREE
HISTORY AND EXAMINATION

A patient presenting to the ENT surgeon with hoarseness or
alteration in voice, has the case history taken and an examination, particular attention is paid to the upper respiratory tract; this is followed by investigations necessary to
confirm the diagnosis. If speech therapy is required, these
steps will precede a joint consultation and referral to the
speech therapist. While the patient is having speech therapy
close cooperation with the ENT surgeon should be maintained by the therapist.

It is necessary to know the duration of the hoarseness and
whether it is persistent or intermittent. The patient is asked
if there are any associated symptoms such as pain or difficulty in swallowing (dysphagia) or earache (otalgia). The
presence of a cough and its nature, whether dry or pro-
ductive, is checked and enquiries are made about the
patient's general health, smoking habits and past medical
history. The social history includes details about the
patient's work, housing, occupation and social use of the
voice.

EXAMINATION

A concave head mirror is used to reflect light on to the
upper respiratory tract and this enables both hands of the
examiner to be free for using instruments. The anterior
nares are examined with a nasal speculum, and the pharynx
with a tongue depressor. A small angled mirror is used to
examine the postnasal space and a larger angled mirror to
examine the larynx. It is important to assess whether the
nasal airway is normal, for nasal obstruction gives a voice
with poor resonance.

43

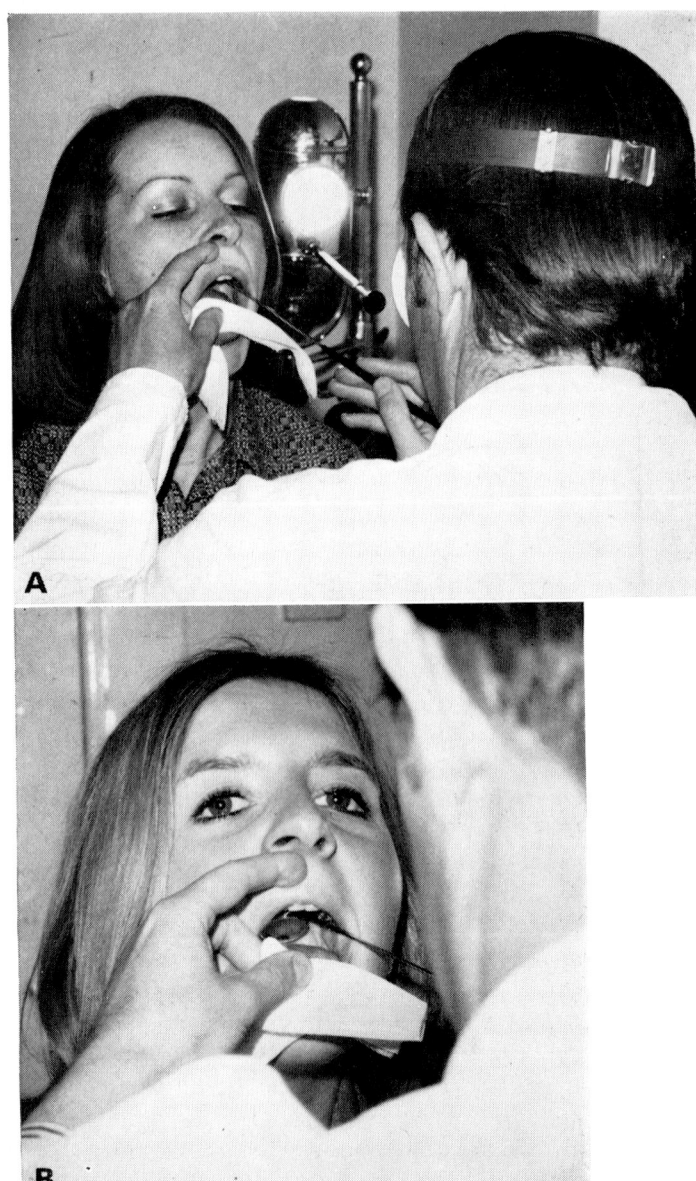

Figure 13 A, Indirect laryngoscopy: B, Position of the laryngeal mirror resting against the soft palate.

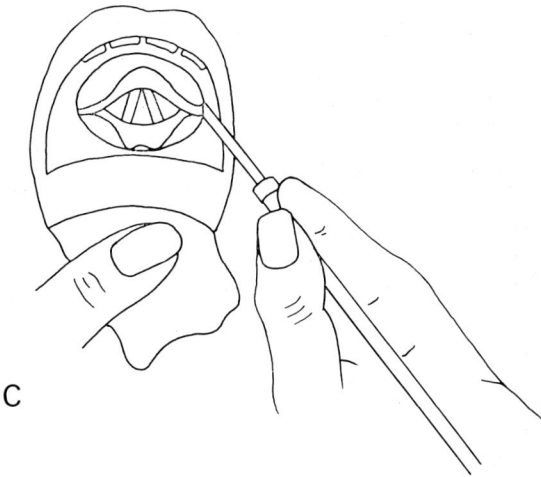

Figure 13   C, The mirror-view of the larynx seen on indirect laryngo-scopy.

Examination of the larynx is uncomfortable for the patient and some voluntary inhibition of the gag reflex is necessary; most adults and some children can achieve this without an anaesthetic spray or lozenge having to be used to reduce the sensitivity of the mucous membrane. Indirect laryngoscopy (Figure 13), although uncomfortable, is not a painful procedure. Dentures, if present, are removed and the patient's tongue is protruded and held with a piece of gauze between the examiner's left thumb and middle finger. The index finger retracts the upper lip. The mirror is warmed to avoid misting and placed at the level of the soft palate. The examiner obtains a clear view of the larynx and surrounding structures and is usually able to demonstrate these to an observer looking over his right shoulder. Patients vary greatly in the anatomy of their tongue, palate and epiglottis and the ease of the examination not only depends on the patient's cooperation but on the size of the tongue and the shape of the epiglottis. The larynx of children under the age of ten is difficult or impossible to see; not only may the child be frightened and uncooperative, but the curved infantile epiglottis obscures a view of the cords. In some cases this 'infantile epiglottis' persists into adult life and this anatomical variant is a factor that may make indirect laryngoscopy impossible in some adults. The larynx of a baby or toddler is rarely visible on indirect laryngoscopy. A clear view of the vocal cords should, however, be obtained in almost every patient presenting with hoarseness. Failure to achieve this usually necessitates a direct laryngoscopy under general anaesthetic. A laryngeal tomogram X-ray frequently gives useful information about a larynx that can not be seen with indirect laryngoscopy and in an adult, this is a common investigation preceding direct examination.

Fibre optic endoscopes are also used for examination of the larynx. A narrow flexible glass fibre tube with a light source is inserted into the nostril and passed back into the postnasal space, local anaesthetic having been applied to the inside of the nose. This technique gives a clear view of the larynx in most cases and is useful in that it may make a direct laryngoscopy unnecessary when the indirect examination is unsuccessful.

These details of history, examination, and investigation are dealt with by the ENT surgeon and if the condition diagnosed requires the further opinion and management of the speech therapist, a joint consultation is arranged. It is then necessary for the speech therapist to take a further case history and examination with attention to details relevant to management.

OUTLINE OF A CASE HISTORY

Speech Therapy

History of present voice problem:	Duration
	Intermittent or persistent
Past history:	Previous voice problem
	Previous speech therapy
Occupation:	Details of work and surroundings
	Amount of voice use
	Noise conditions
	Telephone use
Irritants:	Smoking
	Alcohol
	Dust or chemical irritants (occupation or hobby)

General health: Recurring illnesses, particularly those involving respiratory tract, *e.g.*, asthma, bronchitis
Serious illness or operation
Back trouble
Female patients—details of menstrual cycle
Drugs, tablets
Appetite, sleep

Anxieties, strains or stresses:

Social/family history: Married or single
Family details
Housing details
Hobbies and interests

Details of breathing: Mouth or nose
Snoring
Breathlessness

Weight:

Techniques and Details of Taking the Case History

Before seeing a patient with a voice disorder the speech therapist should read the medical notes. The ENT history and examination and the referring letter from the general practitioner give the preliminary information required prior to taking the history. The therapist's manner and approach are important. Interest in the patient must be evident but not inquisitive. It is usually easier to discuss the more personal problems and worries at the first interview when the patient/therapist relationship is at an impersonal stage. Patients may hedge in their replies and the therapist can then either press for the information by repeating the question or by rephrasing it. Those who say they have no problems or worries may well begin to talk more freely if they are assured that one is not looking for a major crisis which is well remembered, but for a number of minor difficulties. There may be a refusal to answer questions, but this will usually change when it is pointed out that the replies are needed for the assessment and the basis of treatment, and if the information is not given it is much harder for the speech therapist to help.

It is a good plan to let the patient describe in his own words, the onset and history of the present voice difficulty, rather than using a bombardment of direct questions. Most patients may not have been asked to give all the details, due to lack of time in the general practitioner's surgery and in a busy outpatient department, and they find a certain amount of relief in having the opportunity and time to talk more freely. It affords the speech therapist the chance to listen to the voice and so begin the voice assessment and be able to judge the type of patient and case history. The verbose person who gives a plethora of details will need specific questions and firm handling. The aggressive person who will not cooperate will need an explanation of why certain questions are asked so that his cooperation can be obtained.

The patient should be asked for his explanation of the cause, which may prove to be valid. Frequently a linking of the various events that preceded the voice trouble becomes evident.

The occupation is often related to the voice disorder. The amount of talking involved in the patient's job must be considered, as must the degree of background noise. The therapist must ascertain the pressures of the particular job and the responsibilities involved. Because of the importance of posture in voice production it is necessary to obtain details about this. If the patient works in a quiet office with considerable telephone use, it is revealing to learn how the patient sits when taking the calls and it is often quicker to ask the patient to demonstrate rather than describe.

The irritants, smoking and alcohol, are often closely linked. It is interesting to see that the amount of smoking reported to the speech therapist is nearly always in excess of that reported to the surgeon. Questions about drinking may reveal the heavy drinker who is irritating his pharyngeal mucous membrane with neat spirits or the man who, whilst consuming modest amounts of beer, is spending each evening in the hot, smoky atmosphere of a noisy pub. The replies given to the questions on general health may be very indicative of the patient's type. The worrier for example will give many details of minor aches and pains and any operation will be related in detail. A history of repeated attacks of asthma or bronchitis will alert the therapist to pay close attention to the patient's breathing pattern. The terms 'arthritis' and 'rheumatism' may be used somewhat loosely but they will often highlight aches and pains in the neck, shoulders and back which may have affected posture and breathing. Any history of 'back trouble' should be discussed further in order to establish whether this has necessitated wearing a surgical corset, as a garment of this sort may well have interfered with correct breathing. Serious illness or recent operations may have given rise to worry and stress. Sometimes an operation can have altered breathing because of pain and discomfort.

Details regarding the female patient's menstrual cycle may seem far removed from a voice disorder but they are relevant. It is surprising how many women are distressed by dysmenorrhoea but fail to seek advice. The stress involved may well be linked to the voice problem. Some women may have noted voice changes during the menstrual cycle. If the woman has undue premenstrual tension the voice may become more harsh or strident at this time. There may well be more vocal abuse at this stage if shouting and arguing take place because of premenstrual tension. It is necessary to know if the menopause has occurred as this affects the prognosis for the range of voice. Some women are very distressed by hot flushes and hormone tablets may be prescribed which contain an androgen in small quantities and this may have a virilizing effect on the voice. The discussion on the menstrual cycle gives the opportunity to discuss contraceptive problems which may be giving rise to stress.

The question 'do you worry?' is an important one, for it may bring out real problems and worries or merely show that the patient is an inveterate worrier who is always tense over some minor details. It is the question that draws people to talk about themselves. When there is a strong denial of any problem whatsoever it may, in fact, suggest that there are worries that are being concealed or not being faced up to.

Late in the history-taking, one will have an indication of the marital status—whether single or married, widowed, divorced or separated, as the partner will usually have been

mentioned. Inquiries must be made regarding children—
the number and age range. Young children and teenagers
may create problems within a home and so may contribute
to a voice disorder.

If the patient is single, tactful inquiries must be made as to
whether or not they live alone or with a partner of the same
or opposite sex. A homosexual may be subjected to certain
pressures which may have repercussions on a voice problem.

Many hobbies, such as amateur acting or singing, supporting a local football team, involve voice use, frequently
against a noisy background and so it is necessary to learn
about the patient's interests. The person without hobbies or
interests may be finding life somewhat dull and boring.

Details of the breathing habits are important; observation may show that there is mouth-breathing and this can be
verified if the patient has noticed this and a history of snoring will be further confirmation. It is helpful to know if
there is breathlessness on exertion, such as climbing a flight
of stairs; this may reveal a history of minor breathing difficulties which have been increasing. It is better to inquire
about weight at this stage rather than when asking about
health as the apprehensive patient may jump to the conclu-
sion that one suspects a serious illness. So often enquiries
about weight will reveal the patient who has put on weight
after giving up playing some sport.

Management of Voice Production Disorders

The technique and mechanism of correct voice production is
described to the patient and the various factors which may
have caused incorrect voice are pointed out, with an explanation of how the speech therapist proposes to help to
overcome these faults. When dealing with cases of abnormal
voice it is important that the speech therapist is constantly
aware of normal voice. Normal voice depends on expired air
from the lungs being coordinated with phonation, the pitch
being adapted to age and sex. The vocal note produced is
then amplified and modified to give correct voice.

This introduces the question of exercises or practice; since
the speech therapist is dependent on the patient's cooperation, the patient's confidence in speech therapy must be

encouraged. A full explanation of the proposed treatment is given and questions and discussion are encouraged. The therapist must be tactful when pointing out the faults in voice production for no-one likes being told they are doing something incorrectly. Sensitive and resistant patients need particularly careful handling.

It is important to ensure that the patient realizes that the exercises are a means to an end and that unless there is a 'carry-over' from voice exercises to voice production in conversation they are useless. If there is a failure to grasp this concept the exercises may be beautifully and expertly performed, but the voice production in conversation will remain faulty. The patient who is somewhat resistant to realizing that he needs speech therapy will view the exercises with considerable scepticism unless they are closely linked with normal situations and an explanation must be given. It is pointed out that exercises are a drill so that new technique can be mastered. Since one is changing bad habits to good ones, there is a need to concentrate in the early stages on the mechanics of breathing and voice production and so be able to gain such control that in talking, full attention can be paid to what is being said.

The speech therapy exercises should be carried out at least twice daily. There should always be some practice for the patient before starting the day's work so that they have reminded themselves early in the day that voice production needs care. If there are breathing problems, they are asked to think of correct breathing when performing some routine task. The houswife can link this to washing up or housework; the car driver can think of good breathing as he walks to the car and breathing can be corrected. The main practice session should be during the evening after work when the patient has more time available. The exercises should be written down for they are unlikely to be remembered clearly or in the correct order. The directions should be simple and easy to follow, and care should be taken to avoid possible misinterpretation. It is wise to eliminate the term 'breathe in' as most lay people's reaction is to tighten in the diaphragm region. The therapist should ensure that her writing is readable by the patient and should check over the instructions so that the details of the exercises are clear.

This check also ensures that commas are in the right place. the exercises, 'FILL 2,3—OUT 2,3' becomes nearly impossible for most patients if the commas are not in the correct places.

The instructions can be written in a note book but there will probably be waste, for it is unlikely that the treatment will continue until the book is filled. Pieces of paper are easily lost and soon become damaged. An index card, 8×5 in, is a good solution; it is firm enough and can be carried in a handbag or wallet and the patient can prop it up in front of him during practice.

Since voice production is based on posture and relaxation, these must be established first. Exercises can be given to ensure relaxation of neck and shoulders, such as shoulder shrugging or headrolling, though with the latter, care must be taken to ensure it is not attempted too vigorously.

One can then proceed to correct diaphragmatic breathing. This can be difficult to establish if the patient has to wear a surgical corset or because of weight problems wears a firm foundation garment. The 'long-line' bra may also hamper easy breathing.

The emphasis in breathing exercises for voice production is the control of expiration and it is only when this is obtained that resonance work can be started. It is usual to start by humming an easy note, and then to proceed to a hum followed by a vowel sound. The patient should be made aware of the tactile sensation. Some patients become embarrassed by the noises they are asked to make and need reassurance.

Practice should be carefully graded but there must be variety for if the same thing is repeated too frequently it becomes boring and there is loss of interest. Things said by rote are useful in the early work as the patient can concentrate on the expiration of air and the production of voice. Names and addresses are useful as a next step as there is variety and some thinking is required.

Basic Exercises for Voice Production

A *For relaxation of neck and shoulders to establish good posture*

   1 Shrug shoulders in circular movements, forwards and backwards

2 Drop head forward, roll it round slowly once each way—this exercise must be done slowly and easily

B *Breathing exercises*

Hands on ribs, breathe out to fullest limit

1 FILL, HOLD, OUT—three times

2 FILL 2 (seconds), HOLD 2, OUT 2—three times (*i.e.* the same as the first exercise but taken one pace slower)

3 FILL 2,3, HOLD 2,3, OUT 2,3—three times

4 FILL, HOLD, OUT in two even puffs—three times (this helps the patient begin to budget out-going air)

5 FILL, HOLD, OUT slowly, counting to self—four times

6 FILL, HOLD, OUT slowly, counting aloud—four times

C *Resonance work*

1 FILL, HOLD, OUT to easy hum, felt by nose—five times
The patient should use a pitch that is easy to maintain and should be made aware of any alteration of sound which may occur as the air supply runs out

2 Hum, followed by vowel sounds
Mmmm‿AH
Mmmm‿AY, etc.

3 Starting with a hum and proceeding to a day of the week
Mmmm‿Monday
Mmmm‿Tuesday, etc.

4 As above proceeding to months
Mmmm‿January
Mmmm‿February, etc.

5 Days of the week, without a hum

6 Months of year, without a hum

7 Counting in group of numbers, topping up with air inbetween each group, 12, 3,—4, 5, 6—7, 8, 9, etc., gradually increasing the groups of numbers

8 Names and addresses

The above exercises form a basis and can be added to or varied.

Reading aloud for voice work should be suggested with care. Many patients are embarrassed by reading aloud and this will hinder rather than promote good voice production. However, some patients will enjoy reading aloud and this can be incorporated into their practice. Since they are reading for good voice production rather than interest, it is helpful to start with reading aloud, headlines and then proceed to short paragraphs. When good voice production is nearly established, they can be asked to read items of interest.

General conversation practice will be used in the treatment session: at first it will be necessary for the therapist to point out each time poor voice production occurs, but slowly the patient should become aware without a reminder and be able to correct faults. Finally, good voice production should be heard throughout the conversation, even when the subject is one of concern and interest to the patient.

CHAPTER FOUR

LARYNGEAL OPERATIONS

DIRECT LARYNGOSCOPY AND MICROLARYNGOSCOPY

Examination of the larynx is carried out with a laryngoscope inserted through the mouth to a position just above the ventricular bands. Because of the gag and cough reflex and pain of any instrumentation to the larynx, this procedure is carried out under general anaesthetic with a narrow anaesthetic tube placed posteriorly between the cords. Direct laryngoscopy can be managed under local anaesthetic, with surface anaesthetic sprays to the mucosa of the pharynx and larynx, the patient is also given a tranquillizer or sedative.

Direct laryngoscopy enables a thorough examination of the larynx and is necessary if a clear view of the larynx cannot be obtained at indirect laryngoscopy in a patient complaining of hoarseness. There are sites in the larynx where a lesion may not be seen on indirect laryngoscopy and these are examined with particular care on direct laryngoscopy; the ventricle, the subglottic region and the epiglottis just above the anterior commissure (tubercle or petiolus of the epiglottis) are the main concealed sites.

Direct Laryngoscopy with use of the Operating Microscope (Microlaryngoscopy)

The adult vocal cords are about 2 cm in length from the anterior to the posterior commissure and in a baby or toddler or child, the cords are considerably shorter. Only relatively gross anatomy is therefore apparent when the larynx is examined with direct vision through a laryngoscope, the lumen of which is only about 1 to 3 cm in diameter and 17 cm in length. A portion of a large ulcer such as a

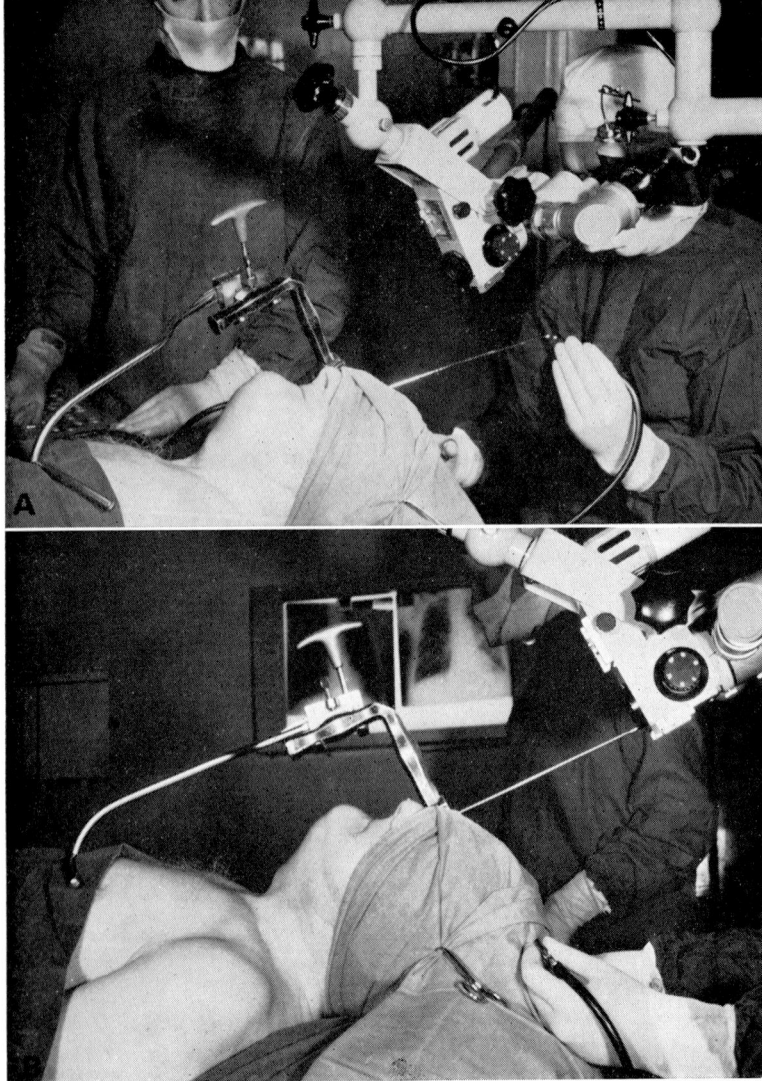

Figure 14   A, Position of the operating microscope (with tutur viewing arm) and the laryngoscope, which is secured with a clamp resting on the patient's chest.   B, The tube delivering oxygen and the anaesthetic, which is not in view, is placed through the nose. The chest X-ray is in the background.

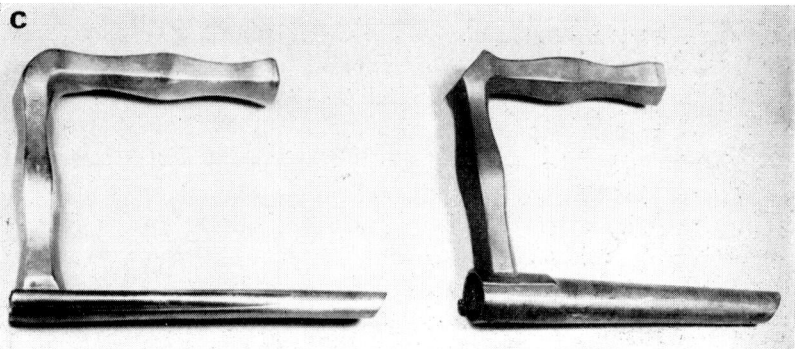

Figure 14   C, Laryngoscopes. The wider laryngoscope on the right is used in microlaryngoscopy.

carcinoma can be taken under direct vision for histological examination or a large polyp readily seen and excised. For detailed examination of the vocal cords, however, and for surgery to the vocal cords, the operating microscope is used. It is placed between the laryngoscope (which is secured to the patient's chest with a holder) and the surgeon (Figure 14). An excellent view of the cords is obtained under magnification and both hands of the surgeon are free to use fine microlaryngeal instruments. This technique is now routine for most endolaryngeal surgery and enables such small lesions as vocal cord nodules or juvenile papillomas to be removed with precision.

An ulcer of the larynx or an area of leukoplakia requires direct laryngoscopy for a portion of this lesion to be removed: this is the biopsy specimen which is sent for microscopic examination. All laryngeal lesions removed at direct laryngoscopy are biopsied so that a definite diagnosis can be made. The operating microscope helps in the accuracy of the taking of the biopsy, so that the tissue is taken from the most suspicious part of the lesion with minimal damage to the surrounding normal structures of the larynx.

Teflon injection of the larynx for treatment of a vocal cord palsy is another procedure that can be carried out with direct laryngoscopy. Teflon, which is a polythene well accepted by the body, with minimal foreign body reaction, is available as a suspension that can be injected. A metal syringe with a long needle is used and about 1 cc of teflon is injected into the laryngeal soft tissue lateral to the immobile cord. The mass of teflon displaces the cord to the mid-line to the point where the normal cord can fully adduct and the ability to close the glottis is restored. In almost all cases there is a dramatic improvement in voice and the cough becomes effective. Teflon injection can also be carried out under local anaesthesia with an indirect laryngoscopy technique. Many cases of idiopathic vocal cord palsy either recover spontaneously or good compensation on adduction is developed by the mobile cord, so that there are few of these cases requiring teflon injection.

TRACHEOSTOMY

Obstruction of the airway at the level of the cords or above, is treated with an opening through the upper rings of the trachea and the insertion of a curved patent tube. Extensive carcinomas, juvenile papillomas and large cysts or polyps may cause respiratory obstruction and stridor. The obstruction may be relatively sudden, requiring an emergency tracheostomy. An inhaled or an impacted foreign body in the larynx may also necessitate an emergency tracheostomy, as may a bilateral cord palsy or rheumatoid cricoarytenoid joint fixation. Once the tracheostomy tube is in place the patient can breathe satisfactorily, but the voice is poor unless the lumen of the tracheostomy tube is temporarily occluded. A valved inner tube is available which lets air in on inspiration and closes on expiration. This is a speaking tube and is useful in restoring voice to patients with a permanent tracheostomy. This may be necessary with juvenile papillomas or following severe trauma to the larynx. Although laryngeal obstruction is the commonest indication for a tracheostomy, it is also carried out for control of respiration with respiratory paralysis, which may be caused by polio, tetanus or drug-overdose coma. The tube into the trachea also enables mucus from the trachea and bronchi to be removed by suction; when the cough reflex is absent or depressed a tracheostomy may therefore be performed for severe pneumonias and also for severe crush injuries to the chest when rib and diaphragm movement is inadequate and control of ventilation with a pump is required.

LARYNGOFISSURE

This operation is now relatively uncommon. In this operation, one vocal cord from the anterior commissure to the vocal process of the arytenoid posteriorly is excised. The larynx is approached by a neck incision to expose the thyroid cartilage. The cartilage is opened vertically in the midline from the notch to the cricothyroid membrane and the alae are retracted laterally. This exposes the interior of the larynx and gives good access to the vocal cords enabling excision of the cord. A temporary tracheostomy is performed while the area where the cord has been excised heals.

The main indication for the laryngofissure was in an early carcinoma of the vocal cord, but modern radiotherapy gives equally good cure rates and has displaced this operation. There is, however, still a place for the laryngofissure; a recurrence of a carcinoma confined to the cord after radiotherapy or residual cord carcinoma after radiotherapy are the main indications. A full course of radiotherapy to the larynx cannot be repeated for the maximum dose is given that will destroy the carcinoma, but not irreversibly damage the adjacent normal tissue of the larynx. Further radiotherapy or an excessive initial dose causes severe inflammatory destruction of the laryngeal cartilages. Inflammation involving cartilage is known as *perichondritis* and the damage to normal tissue caused by excess radiotherapy is *radionecrosis*. A superficial radionecrotic ulcer may remain after treatment of a carcinomatous ulcer with radiotherapy, and a differential diagnosis between a radionecrotic and a residual carcinoma is sometimes difficult, necessitating a biopsy. The laryngofissure is still the operation of choice for a cord carcinoma when modern radiotherapy is not available and the cure rates are similar. A recurrent benign papilloma of the vocal cord which recurs after repeated removal at direct laryngoscopy also may require laryngofissure.

The laryngofissure approach to the larynx is also used to

enable laryngeal cysts, which are too large to be removed via laryngoscope, to be excised. Also, in cases of damage to both recurrent laryngeal nerves, when the airway is impaired, the excision of one arytenoid and fixation of the cord laterally to enlarge the opening of the larynx can be managed via the laryngofissure approach. A tumour that has extended from the vocal cord on to the arytenoid can also be excised by this approach, one type of *partial laryngectomy*, which may prevent a patient having a total laryngectomy. Patients will develop a coherent but hoarse voice after laryngofissure, which is improved with speech therapy, but a normal voice is rarely, if ever, obtained.

The standard of voice varies considerably as it depends on where the scar tissue at the site of the excised cord forms, a matter over which there is little control. If a ridge of scar tissue is on a line with the remaining healthy cord then good compensation can be achieved and the voice, although hoarse, will be strong. If the scar forms above or below the normal cord level there will always be a considerable amount of air waste and the voice will be breathy and lack power.

The aims of speech therapy are good compensation across the mid-line of the glottis by the healthy cord and to help the patient cope with the continual air waste. The first aim is achieved by glottal work and the second by breathing exercises. It is difficult to manage much variety in glottal exercises. Many patients are embarrassed by the noises they are asked to make but the patient should be made aware that the speech therapist realizes the crudeness of the sounds she is requesting. Pushing exercises may be used and are particularly helpful in the early stages. Pushing against a heavy piece of furniture or the wall is effective to produce an audible glottal stop at the end of each push. The exercises need not be done too vigorously since these patients need to replenish air frequently; upper chest breathing can be encouraged and they should be made aware of the effect of air loss on vocal quality. A good degree of nasal resonance will give the voice greater carrying power. One of the early signs of recurrence of the carcinoma is deterioration of voice and the speech therapist must be alert to any voice change. When the patient is attending on a review basis it is helpful to both surgeon and therapist if there is a tape-recording available for reference.

TOTAL LARYNGECTOMY

Total laryngectomy is necessary for most cases of carcinoma of the larynx that have not been cured with radiotherapy. Patients with extensive supra- and subglottic laryngeal carcinomas when first seen, may have a disease that is so advanced that the likelihood of cure with radiotherapy is very small; in these cases, laryngectomy is carried out and radiotherapy may not be used.

There are very rare instances when a laryngectomy is carried out for conditions other than carcinoma. Extensive infection and breakdown of the larynx due to perichondritis following radiotherapy may leave the patient almost voiceless with a painful larynx and a tracheostomy: this situation may necessitate laryngectomy. Laryngectomy has also been carried out on rare occasions for gross neuromuscular incoordination of swallowing in which 'spill' of saliva and food into the trachea and bronchi causes recurrent pneumonia.

A total laryngectomy is made through a U-shaped incision in the neck; the skin is elevated to expose the underlying laryngeal cartilages and muscles. The larynx from above the hyoid bone to the third or fourth ring of the trachea is excised, the mucous membrane of the pyriform fossae which remains is sutured in the mid-line anteriorly and to the mucosa of the base of the tongue, so that a continuous tube of mucous membrane is formed to reconstruct the pharynx. The trachea is sutured to the skin, so that a laryngectomy patient has a permanent tracheostome just below the collar line (Figure 15). It is often necessary to excise the lobe of the thyroid gland on the side of the carcinoma of the larynx, particularly with subglottic carcinoma. The thyroid gland is closely related to the larynx and direct infiltration of tumour into the gland is not uncommon.

With some laryngeal carcinomas, spread to the neck lymph nodes on the side of the tumour may have occurred. The neck of every patient with laryngeal carcinoma is carefully palpated; if hard, firm, non-tender nodes are felt, it is necessary to remove these lymph nodes with the larynx. This is called a radical neck dissection, or a block dissection

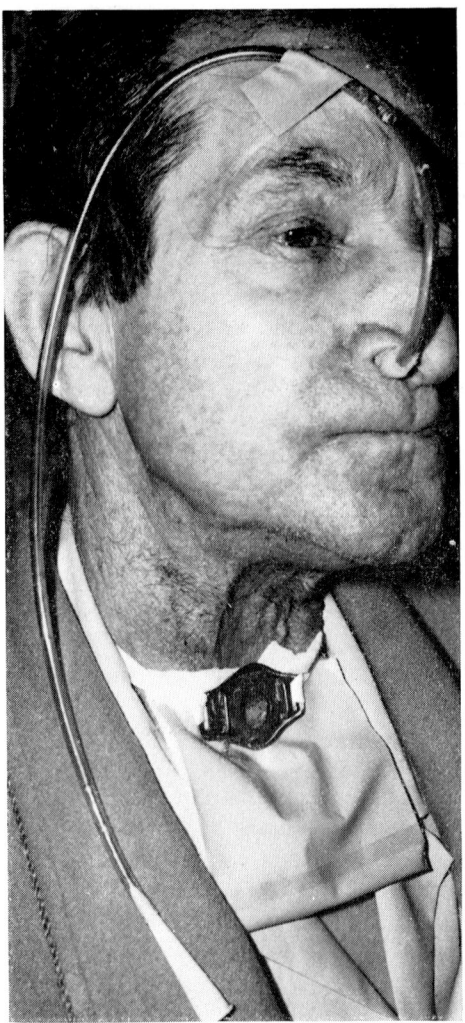

Figure 15 A patient one week following laryngectomy. The skin sutures from the upper part of the 'U'-shaped neck incision have been removed. The feeding tube, which is still in place, is usually removed between the 7th and 14th postoperative day, providing skin healing is good, without evidence of a salivary fistula.

of the cervical lymph glands. The internal jugular vein along which the deep cervical nodes are placed, is removed from the clavicle to the jugular foramen of the base of the skull and the sternomastoid muscle is also completely excised. A laryngectomy is, therefore, associated with a neck dissection if nodes are involved; if the laryngeal carcinoma is large and the nodes are not palpable, a *prophylactic neck dissection* is often carried out, for the probability of small deposits of carcinoma being present in the glands which cannot be felt, is high. A neck dissection with laryngectomy involves considerably more extensive and prolonged surgery than a total laryngectomy alone and there is more postoperative disability to the patient. Despite the extent of the surgery, however, the eventual postoperative disability of a neck dissection is surprisingly small; a weakness of the shoulder for lifting and carrying is the main complaint, because the accessory cranial nerve (XI) is divided and the powerful trapezius muscle is deprived of its main nerve supply.

The hypoglossal nerve may be adherent and involved in secondary carcinoma of the neck: during a radical neck dissection it may therefore be necessary to divide this nerve. A paralysis of the muscle on that side of the tongue follows and this causes some disability as articulation is affected. The patient may have difficulty in the initial stages of swallowing and articulation may be further distorted by the pooling of saliva on the affected side.

During laryngectomy a soft polythene or rubber feeding tube is inserted through the nose and via the reconstructed pharynx into the oesophagus and into the stomach, at the time of operation and the pharyngeal mucosa is sutured round this tube (Figure 16). For about ten to fourteen days the patient is fed via this nasogastric tube. When the tube is removed, normal swallowing is resumed. Most laryngectomies are performed on patients who have had previous radiotherapy. Although there is little to see in the neck skin of a patient following radiotherapy, other than a slight brown pigmentation, the tissues deep to the skin are initially extremely friable and vascular and after some months become firm and scarred with a diminished blood supply. The healing of tissues following radiotherapy is slower than normal tissue. Not infrequently, after laryngectomy, the

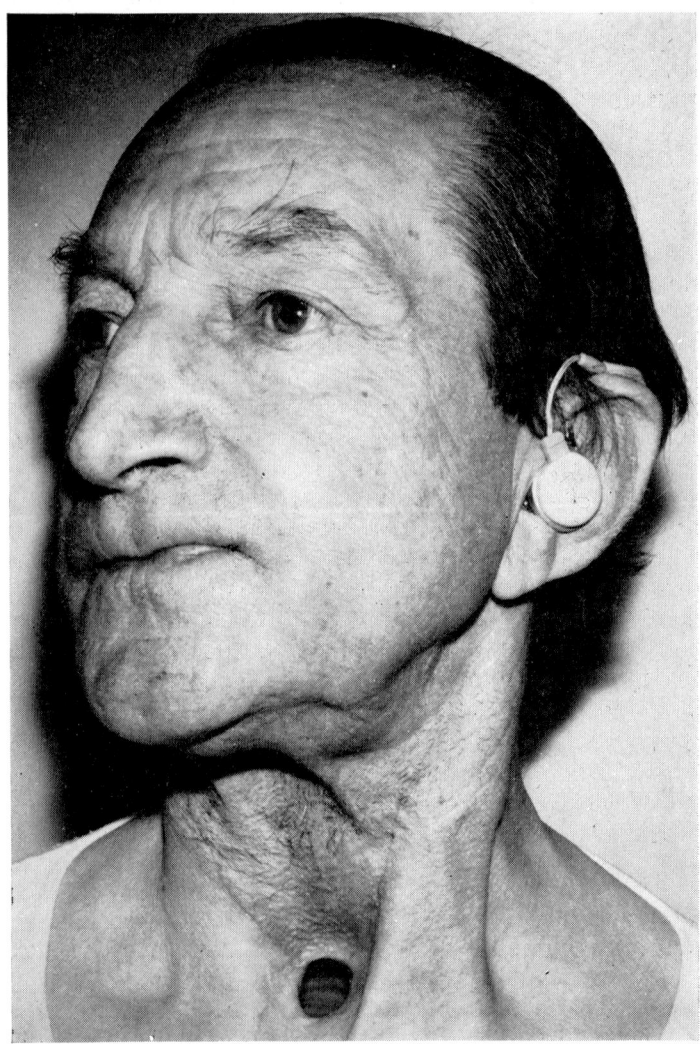

Figure 16 A patient shortly after removal of the feeding tube. All skin sutures have been removed and the 'U'-shaped neck incision is well healed. The rings of the trachea are seen through the tracheostome. Speech therapy is started at this time and it is important for the therapist to be aware of the patient's hearing acuity: this patient's hearing aid is therefore significant to the therapist.

mucosa of the reconstructed pharynx breaks down at one point allowing saliva to track outwards to the skin. These salivary fistula tend to form just above the tracheostome. A salivary fistula heals spontaneously in almost all cases and further surgical closure is usually not required. Healing may, however, take several weeks; these weeks are very frustrating for the patient because a nasogastric tube is uncomfortable and the tube is not removed and normal swallowing cannot be resumed until the fistula has closed.

After the removal of the nasogastric tube, speech therapy for the development of a pharyngeal or oesophageal voice can be started. If speech therapy is started too soon after pharyngeal healing, it is possible that forcing air into the newly healed pharynx may cause the mucous membrane to break down with recurrence of the fistula. The speech therapist must guard against the patient 'forcing' in the pharynx during the early stages of learning pseudo-voice. It is also important that the permission of the medical and nursing staff have been given to the speech therapist before speech therapy work is started.

SPEECH THERAPY FOR THE LARYNGECTOMY PATIENT

The speech therapist plays a major part in the rehabilitation of laryngectomy patients and the acquisition of pseudo-voice facilitates the return to everyday life. It is important that the speech therapist realizes that the aim is not solely that of helping the patient to achieve pseudo-voice, for concern with the person as a whole and interest in the individual is important. Much can be done to ease the acceptance of the disability involved in this type of operation. Morale is often extremely low in these patients. They may be embarrassed by their appearance and this problem is particularly marked in women who have undergone laryngectomy. There is certainly frustration and irritation with the difficulty in communication.

The speech therapist should be conversant with the details of the laryngectomy operation. This would include knowing whether it has been combined with neck dissection and whether the type and extent of the laryngeal cancer favoured a good prognosis.

Pseudo-voice

The aim in trying to produce a pseudo-voice is to charge air into the oesophagus and to utilize the noise that is made on its return. There are three principle methods of air-charging:

1 Swallowing
2 Inspiration
3 Injection

Swallowing Most patients find that they produce a noise when they belch. If there is no speech therapy service available patients will develop this further and their method of 'voice' production will depend on deliberately swallowing air. There are certain disadvantages in this method; firstly there is a time lag between the swallow and the return of air and secondly, it is not easy to control the speed of the returning air. A further disadvantage can be that not all the air is returned and this can give discomfort and a feeling of indigestion and may lead to flatulence. This method, however, is employed inadvertently by all patients in that a certain amount of air is swallowed while eating and this air will return later, probably when they start to talk. It is the use of this swallowed air that gives the rather loud bursts of pseudo-voice that occur shortly after eating.

Inspiration In this method, patients are deliberately taught to synchronize air-charging into the oesophagus and inspiration of air into the lungs via the stoma and then to coordinate the expiration of air from the lungs and oesophagus. This certainly helps achieve smoothness of 'voice' but it has the disadvantage of drawing the patient's attention to his altered breathing mechanism.

Injection The tongue, lips and cheeks are used to help push the air into the oesophagus or its substitute, the air is taken to approximately the level of the cricopharyngeus and then returned with sound. It is the method favoured by most speech therapists.

The speech therapy work with laryngectomized patients divides into three stages and each one is equally important. These stages are:

Preoperative work
Postoperative work
Voice work

Preoperative A preoperative visit is usually requested by the surgeon as it is felt that the speech therapist should have the opportunity to explain about the new method of voice production. If there is a good relationship between the nursing staff and the speech therapist then the former will use this visit to verify that the patient has grasped the essential details of what is involved in this type of operation; the loss of the normal means of voice and a permanent opening in the neck. It is not the speech therapist's task to make the patient aware of these points but if it becomes apparent that there has been a misunderstanding about the nature of the operation or that there is some confusion, the medical staff can be informed and a further explanation given. Few patients understand fully that they will be completely voiceless temporarily after the operation. They usually think that they will have some sort of whisper.

Proper counselling preoperatively can reduce distress in the immediate postoperative stage. It is also wise to confirm that the patient's ability to read and write has not been overlooked. The speech therapist uses this visit to give an explanation of the new type of voice production and when this can be started. It should be remembered that the patient will probably be anxious so that the explanation should be as *brief* and simple as possible. An excess of detailed information to someone already understandably anxious about the operation is frequently harmful and confusing. Some simple diagrams of the present and future voice mechanisms may also prove helpful. Questions about the new voice may well be asked and points clarified that have not been fully understood. Various points may also be raised that the patient has not liked to trouble the surgeon with; such as whether it will still be possible to wear a collar and tie.

One of the important reasons for the preoperative visit is

that the speech therapist can make an assessment of the patient's speech standards and so make a prognosis of the standard of pseudo-voice that may be achieved if this is acquired. The better the articulation and the larger the vocabulary, the greater will be the likelihood of a desire to produce a good pseudo-voice, as unobtrusive as possible, and a great effort for quiet air-charging to reduce stoma noise will be made. Those with poor slovenly articulation and a limited vocabulary will be content with a lower standard of pseudo-voice and they will not be upset by stoma noise or by noisy air-charging. It is fruitless to try to force the patient to try to achieve a higher standard of communication than was present preoperatively.

If an accent or dialect is apparent, it is helpful to note this for it makes lip reading in the early postoperative stage easier. It should be remembered that it is often difficult to establish a good therapist/patient relationship at this visit as the patient is under considerable stress. There will have been meetings with a large number of the hospital staff, such as nurses on the ward, members of the surgical team, physiotherapist and social workers. Visits to the X-ray department will have been made and blood samples taken. The patient may become anxious and confused by the number of hospital staff visits. The overseas patient may present problems if there is no mutual language. It is possible to work with an interpreter but care must be taken so that it can be ensured the interpreter is well conversant with both languages involved. A smattering of English will not suffice to explain the new voice mechanism.

When it comes to the 'voice' work stage, it is possible to work without an interpreter; the patient can be requested to imitate the therapist and produce voice this way. It is not the most satisfactory method, but is possible.

Postoperative   It may not be possible for the speech therapist to visit the patient in the intensive care unit and the first postoperative visit is made on return to the open ward. These visits may seem to be a type of social visit but they serve several purposes. A better patient/therapist relationship can be established and the therapist can learn about the patient's interests and hobbies so that these can be talked about when the voice work is being carried out. Perhaps the greatest benefit of these visits is that they reassure the patient that something will be done about 'voice' and that the matter is under control. There is the opportunity of communicating with somebody who fully understands the problems of lack of voice and the difficulty in talking. If home visitors are few and on a busy ward, there may be little apparent time for conversation and this may give rise to a feeling of isolation for the patient. The therapist's visits give further opportunities of discussing the new voice mechanism and asking any questions.

The patient should be encouraged in this early stage to 'mouth' rather than communicate by writing only. The use of mouthing not only ensures that there is maximum mobility of the tongue, lips and cheeks and that articulation is well under control, it also reinforces the idea that 'voice' communication will follow at the appropriate stage.

Voice work   This is not usually started until the nasogastric feeding tube has been removed. It is wise to wait until the patient has had two feeds by mouth, for a fistula or signs of one will have become apparent in this time. If voice work has been started and a fistula develops necessitating reinsertion of the feeding tube, the patient invariably associates voice work with the breakdown. When voice work is recommenced at a later stage there is an understandable reluctance and preference to remain silent rather than risk further fistula formation.

It is unwise to treat on the open ward when working on voice. The sensitive patient may well be embarrassed by the strange noises requested in the early stages and may inhibit them rather than have others in the ward listen. Usually, the ward staff will see that a quiet room is available such as sister's office, a side ward or treatment room. It does not worry the patient if members of the hospital staff enter for he assumes that staff will be familiar with the noises the speech therapist is asking him to make.

The patient should be seated in an upright chair so that good posture can be obtained and maintained. If attention is given to posture, it will ensure that there is sufficient relaxation, although there will need to be constant reminders. It also draws attention away from the neck as well as helping to maintain easy rhythmic breathing. Stoma noise will be at a minimum if breathing is steady. The patient can then be asked to air-charge using whichever method the speech therapist favours.

Generally the plosive sounds lead more readily to production of 'voice' for patients in these early stages, in particular 'p' and 'b', so that the initial words to teach are those such as 'pop', 'bob' and 'beer'. There is a need for continual reminders to take more air in so that sound can be obtained. Having achieved single words, progress is made to short phrases, such as, 'pint of beer', 'bread and butter', 'piece of cake'. It is also important to keep reminding the patient to air-charge; it should be stressed that the request is to take air into the throat, but to avoid swallowing. Firmly indicating the level to which the air is to be taken is helpful so that there is a specific point for the patient to aim at.

Opinions vary on the question of giving lists of practice words to be tried between treatment sessions. Frequently, one finds the pseudo-voice is produced on the practice words but that replies to questions are still mouthed or written. It should be remembered that morale is often low at this stage and lists of words may suggest a school room atmosphere. We have found that if the patient is asked to try saying words with the new 'voice', practice with more varied material will develop. It can be suggested that names of members of the family, including pets, objects in the ward, days, months, etc., are used. The aim is for frequent short practices; a long session will tire the patient so that 'voice' is not obtained and a feeling of depression ensues. It is essential, however, to keep assuring the patient that the more 'voice' is used the smoother and easier it will eventually become.

During the treatment time, conversation can be introduced so that the voice is used in a more normal manner. While the patient is in hospital, treatment is once or twice daily. The frequency of visits as an outpatient is often controlled by the travelling time involved.

Failure to Develop Pseudo-voice

There are several reasons underlying the failure to achieve pseudo-voice. The speech therapist should always be on the alert for a possible sign of recurrence and it must be remembered that recurrence of the carcinoma is not an uncommon reason for failure to develop pseudo-voice. When voice is obtained, but there is failure to develop, although the patient is cooperative and following instructions, or it is noticed that there are swallowing difficulties, this may also suggest the possibility of recurrence. Sometimes patients will not trouble the surgeon for mild pain and discomfort but it is mentioned to the speech therapist, who should let the surgeon know. Other reasons for failure to develop pseudo-voice are a positive dislike of the new voice by either the patient or the family; hearing loss so that instructions are not fully grasped and the sounds that are to be made are misunderstood, or lack of motivation found in those who live alone are other factors related to failure. There may be difficulty in accepting and coming to terms with all that the operation has entailed so that there is little devotion and concentration of energy on voice work. There may be emotional or financial family problems that absorb the patient's time and effort.

It is during the visits following discharge that the speech therapist can do so much in helping with rehabilitation. Encouragement to wear a collar and tie to improve the interest of appearance and self-esteem is a typical, small contributory point. Discussion with the wife/husband and family, can ensure that the patient once again fits into the household and begins to lead a more normal life.

Demonstration of another laryngectomy patient   It is important that there should be very careful thought and planning if the new patient is introduced to an 'old' laryngectomy patient. Certain standards must be laid down and maintained, or the visit may be a failure. The demonstrator must have good pseudo-voice and be easily understood. An appearance of fitness is necessary and it is preferable if the patient has returned to work. If the demonstrator is male, he should be wearing a collar and tie and if female, some neat covering over the stoma that matches whatever else is being worn. It is unsatisfactory for the new patient to see a demonstrator who has his stoma completely exposed, who looks ill and is unlikely to return to work. It should be remembered that hearing pseudo-voice for the first time can be a shock, for however good it may be, it does not sound 'normal'. The new patient who has never heard or seen someone who has undergone a laryngectomy may find it very distressing and may make him reconsider giving consent to the operation. Many have been in hospital before for direct laryngoscopy and have seen other patients on the ward who have just started acquiring voice, but may never have heard a well-established pseudo-voice; they will find it encouraging to see a good speaker preoperatively. Some new patients prefer to see a good speaker after the operation rather than before. The voice achieved by a long-term laryngectomee, may range from merely adequate, to one generally acceptable by society in that it attracts little, if any, attention. The 'voice' acquired following pharyngo-laryngectomy, whether using a stomach or colonic pull-up, or neck or chest flap reconstruction, will never achieve the high standards possible after a laryngectomy. It is therefore important when demonstrating to a pharyngolaryngectomy patient, not to use a laryngectomy patient.

Life after Laryngectomy

The prognosis for survival following laryngectomy is good. Carcinoma frequently remains confined to the larynx or neck glands and spread to other parts of the body is not common. The site and extent of the tumour and whether there is palpable spread to the cervical lymph nodes obviously influences the prognosis. The type of carcinoma also influences the prognosis; the biopsy specimen is examined and certain types of tumour are known to have a greater tendency to spread than others. A well-differentiated squamous cell carcinoma tends to remain localized whereas a poorly differentiated or anaplastic carcinoma tends to spread early to the lymphatics or bloodstream.

Most laryngectomy patients learn to acquire a coherent voice with speech therapy. Men, who develop the necessary expertise of injecting air, can produce a near-normal male voice with good volume and control. Women, however, have greater difficulty in accepting the new voice because it is deep and non-feminine. The presence of a permanent opening in the neck is unsettling to many patients and it takes time to adjust to this altered anatomy. Most men patients find that they can wear a collar and tie as they did previously, as a cover for the stoma. They may prefer to wear a gauze bib underneath to absorb a sudden expulsion of mucus to prevent soiling their shirt. Female patients may need some guidance on suitable stoma coverings; a lace cravat can be fashioned with a backing of gauze which can be removed and changed. The cravat can fasten at the back of the neck. Polo neck sweaters and dresses can be worn comfortably. Patients frequently attach a bib pocket on the inside of the polo neck so that staining by coughing is prevented. Heavy necklaces and pendants can also be used, but beads are obviously unwise, for if they break, there is a risk of inhalation into the tracheostome.

The laryngectomy operation is a major operation and there is severe psychological upset to the patient, who requires considerable supportive treatment during rehabilitation. This responsibility comes heavily on to the speech therapist, who sees the patient frequently during the early months following surgery. Not only is the learning of pseudo-voice a difficult challenge to the patient, but the need to adapt breathing through a tracheostome with the altered cough is not easy and many complain of their embarrassment with the cough. Taste and smell are frequently impaired and of course smoking with inhalation is no longer possible. It is also said that the power to lift and cope with heavy work is impaired because of the inability to close the glottis; it is probable, however, that this is not a significant practical factor. Twenty-five postlaryngectomy patients who were examined found little or no difficulty in lifting a 25 lb weight and those who returned to their previous job involving heavy lifting did not complain of altered ability with handling weights. Swimming is also to be avoided and care has to be taken in showers or in the bath that water does not enter the tracheostome. The cough reflex is still strong from the nerve supply to the trachea and bifurcation of the trachea (carinal reflex), and mucus and dust can be readily expelled with the cough.

At laryngectomy, care is taken to fashion the tracheo-stome so that it has an adequate lumen for breathing. Occasionally, however, scar tissue at the junction of the skin and mucous membrane forms causing narrowing, and some patients need to wear a permanent laryngectomy tube to maintain a wide tracheostome. Small plastic studs or buttons are also available and are cleaner and more aesthetic

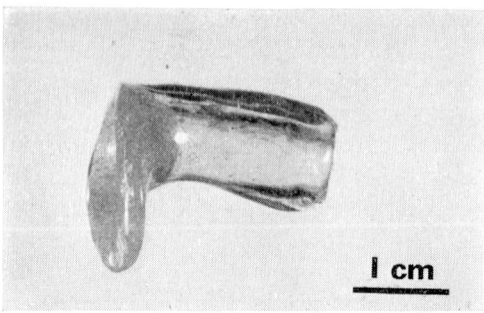

Figure 17 Narrowing of the tracheostome is not uncommon, and a small plastic stud may be preferable to a larger metal laryngectomy tube (Figure 5).

(Figure 17). These are fashioned to fit the tracheostome and are easily inserted; the fibrous ring serves to hold the stud at its neck and keep it in place during conversation and coughing. Crusting of mucus at the tracheostome may also be a problem and a further disturbing factor to the patient.

PHARYNGOLARYNGECTOMY

With carcinoma of the pyriform fossa and upper oeso-phagus, radiotherapy carries a relatively poor cure rate. Laryngectomy associated with removal of the pyriform fossa and upper oesophagus is usually necessary.

If a pyriform fossa tumour is small, there may be sufficient mucosa from the uninvolved pyriform fossa for primary reconstruction of the pharynx and the postoperative situa-tion is similar to the laryngectomy. With carcinomas of the

upper oesophagus (postcricoid carcinomas) and large pyriform fossa carcinomas, however, it is necessary to remove
the pharynx from the base of the tongue to the thoracic inlet,
as well as the larynx—a pharyngolaryngectomy. Replace-
ment and reconstruction of the pharynx involves extensive
and complex surgery (Figure 18). The stomach may be
mobilized through an abdominal incision and brought
through the thorax to suture to the base of the tongue
('stomach pull up'); a segment of the colon, too, can be
mobilized and while still attached to its blood supply brought

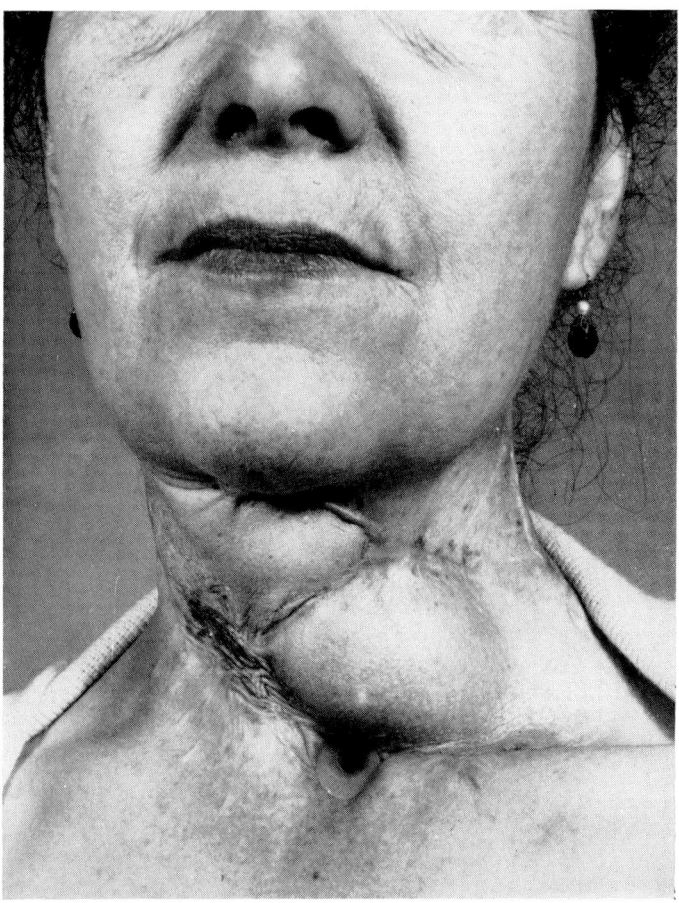

Figure 18   A patient following pharyngolaryngectomy for a carcinoma
of the pyriform fossa, with reconstruction using neck skin flaps.

through the thorax to link to the upper end of the pharynx, while the distal end is linked to the stomach (colon transplant). A third alternative is use of neck and thoracic skin flaps. Following pharyngolaryngectomy, the patient is left with a pharyngostome and oesophagostome, which are to be linked. Neck skin can be raised into flaps that are tubed and used to link the pharyngostome to the oesophagostome and reconstruct the pharynx for swallowing.

In a pharyngolaryngectomy the cricopharyngeus muscle is removed, whereas this muscle is preserved with laryngectomy. The cricopharyngeus enables the patient to develop good control of air released from the pharynx for speech and when this muscle is removed, there is therefore less likelihood of developing good voice and an excellent voice is never achieved.

There are some patients following laryngectomy or pharyngolaryngectomy who are unable to develop speech. A technique has been developed for these patients in which a narrow skin-lined tube is fashioned surgically, extending from the tracheostome to the base of the tongue (Assai technique). Impressive voice production has been demonstrated with this operation, but although an effective surgical technique for some cases, the skin has frequently been irradiated and tends to scar so that the tube closes. It may also break down giving a salivary fistula. This technique has, however, a present-day place for some laryngectomy cases.

During the last decade a number of different surgical procedures have been devised to convey air from the trachea into the oesophagus to ensure pseudo-voice. Assai and his colleagues were the leaders in this field and other surgeons in this field have adapted and modified their procedure. A valved silicone rubber prosthesis has also been used to convey air forced from the lungs into the oesophagus (Edwards, 1974). Modifications are however continuing to be made to the surgical procedure and to the prosthesis, but a standard successful technique has yet to be developed. Taub and his colleagues (1974) have also used a device to be implanted into the neck tissue into which air from the

EDWARDS, N. (1974) *J. Laryngology,* LXXXVIII, **10**, Oct, 905–918.
TAUB, S. (1974) Voice prosthesis for speech restoration in laryngectomies, *Trans. Am. Acad. Ophthalmol. Otolaryngol.,* **78**, 1287–8.

oesophagus is directed to produce sound, this is used to establish audible communication. Speech therapists working with laryngectomized patients must keep in touch with the new surgical procedures developed by the ENT surgeons with whom they work. At the moment they are being developed and perfected, but if they are successful then the role of the speech therapists with laryngectomized patients will be radically altered and have to be reconsidered. The laryngectomized patients will still require help with the problem of rehabilitation and it is interesting to speculate whether the speech therapists should, or could, fulfil this role.

It must be remembered that rarely some patients following laryngectomy do not wish to speak and surgery for this type of patient obviously will not succeed. It is important, there-fore, to exclude this psychological factor in a patient who fails to talk following laryngectomy and for whom the Assai technique is being considered.

Artificial voice aids   Artificial voice aids are also available to those who are unable to develop good pseudo-voice.

Aids produce an artificial sound, as the name implies but their use is considerably better than total silence and it means that voice communication is restored. Most aids tend how-ever to produce a sepulchral or dalek-like tone to which the patient and those listening need to adapt, for the initial response to the artificial voice may be one of alarm.

The oldest type of aid is the reed variety which is based upon the use of air from the stoma activating a reed and the vibra-ting column of air being taken into the corner of the mouth. It is not easy to keep clean, but the sound produced is acceptable. This is not a sophisticated piece of machinery so that mechanical defects are not likely to occur. It is still used in developing countries where there is no speech therapy service and the patient may be illiterate. The 'buzzer' type of aid supplies an external source of noise which transmits vibration of air within the oesophagus and pharynx via a vibrating diaphragm at the head of the buzzer. This is placed by the patient against the neck tissue and so the sound is transmitted. Care has to be taken to find the most suitable place on the neck to put the buzzer (Figure 19). If the neck is

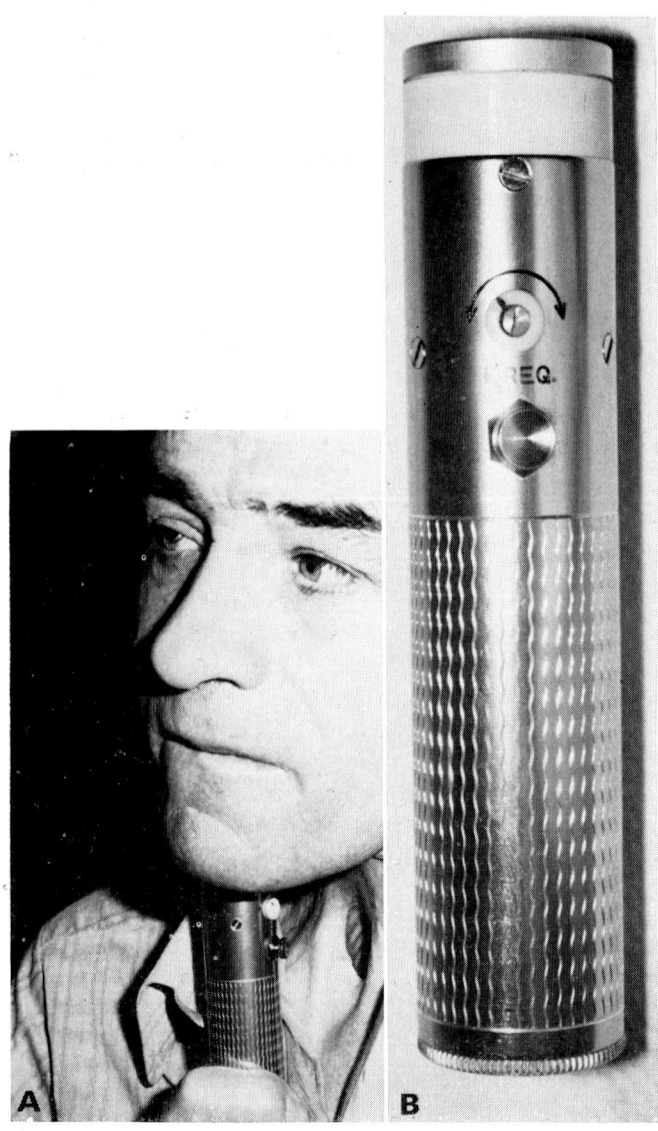

Figure 19   Artificial larynx. This is pressed on the skin under the chin and makes a 'mouthed whisper' clearly audible.

painful, or there is a lot of scarring, patients can find this type of aid most uncomfortable.

The other alternative is an amplifier; a small hand microphone is held close to the mouth and the patient articulates into a small amplifying unit. This type of aid will amplify oesophageal voice as well as mouthing. It must be remembered that patients will need instruction and practice to gain maximum benefit from these aids, whichever type is chosen and the speech therapist will be responsible for assisting the patient after the aid is supplied. In many hospitals, the aid is issued by the hospital and loaned to the patient.

Many speech therapists have strong views about encouraging the use of artificial aids. Personal bias however should not be involved and each case should be assessed according to the factors involved.

Indications for an aid are:

1 Presence of secondaries
   a Those presenting before 'voice' has been established
   b Those presenting a short while after 'voice' has developed and thereby causing its loss
2 Presence of a deaf partner who is unable to hear 'voice'
3 Those patients, or their families, who totally reject 'voice' as being inadequate or repulsive
4 Those patients whose jobs demand talking against background noise

CHAPTER FIVE

SOME CONDITIONS OF THE UPPER RESPIRATORY TRACT AND EAR

Tonsils and Adenoids

Tonsils and adenoids cause problems when recurrent infections or enlargement occur; not infrequently infection and enlargement coexist. The lymphoid tissue in the postnasal space, the adenoids, is present at birth, and is at its maximum size between the ages of three and six. Regression normally occurs after the age of seven and by puberty, little lymphoid tissue remains. It is extremely rare for adenoids to persist after puberty into adult life, so that adenoids rarely cause symptoms after puberty. The adenoids cause nasal and aural symptoms in childhood.

A large pad of adenoids will occlude the posterior choanae of the nose and cause partial or complete nasal obstruction. The child mouth-breathes and snores. There is a characteristic open-mouthed appearance and the voice is often described as 'nasal'. The voice is lacking in resonance and the voice of nasal obstruction is called rhinolalia clausa, or hyporhinophonia. It is important to distinguish this voice from the voice of a child who, because of a short palate or submucosal cleft, is unable to close the postnasal space. The soft palate does not abut against the posterior wall of the pharynx and the voice is altered because air escapes through the nose (rhinolalia aperta, or hyperrhinophonia). This child has difficulty in saying some sounds, particularly 's' which becomes a nasal 'snort'. If an error is made in the diagnosis of this speech problem and removal of adenoids advised for a child with a rhinolalia aperta, there will be an increased escape of air and the voice will be worse. Careful analysis of the voice must therefore precede the decision to remove a child's adenoids for 'nasal' speech. The speech therapist is frequently involved prior to the removal of tonsils and adenoids in the preoperative assessment of the speech. The deviant sounds should be noted and attention given to whether the breathing is through the nose or mouth. The mother should be asked again for details about heavy breathing and snoring; although the surgeon has asked about these the mother may have been hasty and inaccurate in her replies in a busy outpatient department; details are often more forthcoming when the parent has had time to consider a question. The speech therapist will need to know details of eating habits as this will often give an indication of the degree of mouth-breathing. Mouth-breathers tend to be in one of two categories as regards eating—the 'bolters' and the 'slow'. The former 'gulp' their food, whereas the latter are so slow that the food becomes cold and unpalatable and is left and they are often 'faddy' eaters, disliking anything which requires chewing. If the speech therapist finds a history of altered eating habits, it should be mentioned to the surgeon, as it may be a relevant factor to be considered when deciding future management.

Adenoids may also interfere with the function of the Eustachian tube and predispose to attacks of middle ear infection (otitis media). Large adenoids may alter Eustachian tube function so that the middle ear is inadequately ventilated and an accumulation of sterile fluid forms in the middle ear causing deafness (secretory otitis media). This is a very common cause of deafness in children; the middle ear fluid is tenacious and the condition is commonly known as 'glue ear'. Since hearing is so important to the child's development of speech and language the standard of speech and the child's use of language needs to be given attention.

Because of the natural regression of the bulk of adenoids, there is a conservative attitude to their removal. Only if the nasal or aural problems are severe and persistent is adenoidectomy necessary.

Recurrent attacks of acute tonsillitis are the main indication for tonsillectomy. On occasions the bulk of lymphoid tissue of the tonsils causes symptoms in children. Difficulty in swallowing and obstruction to breathing may occur. Tonsils that meet or nearly meet in the mid-line cause an alteration in speech in which the tone is altered. Breathing tends to be noisy and poorly controlled and the obstruction

in the pharynx causes poor resonance and vocal quality·
Articulation tends to lack definition and crispness. As with
removal of adenoids, a conservative attitude is taken with
tonsillectomy. The bulk of the tonsil lymphoid tissue re-
gresses with age and removal of tonsils for symptoms caused
by their size is not as common as removal for recurrent
tonsillitis. It is arguable whether the adjective 'large' can be
correctly applied to tonsils for there is no recognized normal
size (Figure 20). Although tonsils that meet in the mid-line
are abnormal the size may be deceptive. When the tongue is
forcibly protruded or on gagging, there is a tendency for the
fauces to be drawn towards the mid-line so that the tonsils
appear to meet. Whereas when the mouth is opened in a
relaxed way the tonsils are widely separated.

Acute tonsillitis may be complicated by pus forming in the
parapharyngeal space lateral to the tonsil; this is called a
quinsy or a parapharyngeal abscess. It is an extremely
painful condition with malaise, severe dysphagia and earache. A quinsy is rare in children, although not uncommon
in adults. A quinsy is another indication for tonsillectomy
when the acute infection has settled. Both tonsillitis and
quinsy formation are not infrequently associated with
glandular fever (infectious mononucleosis).

Particularly careful preoperative assessment is needed
before the tonsils and adenoids are removed from a child
who has undergone surgical repair of a cleft palate, or who
has a submucous palatal cleft. The palate in these children is
frequently less mobile and shorter than normal so that its
ability to butt against the posterior wall of the oropharynx
and seal the postnasal space is impaired. The bulk of the
adenoid and tonsil lymphoid tissue may in fact assist in this
closure. If tonsils and adenoids are removed, particularly
the adenoids, the ability of the soft palate to seal the postnasal space may be lost, so that the speech becomes worse
postoperatively. The scarring of the fauces which may also
occur after tonsillectomy further limits palatal movement
and accentuates the speech defect.

Children with cleft palates also have impaired Eustachian
tube function, and infection from the nose and postnasal
space (as in head colds) frequently spreads to the middle ear

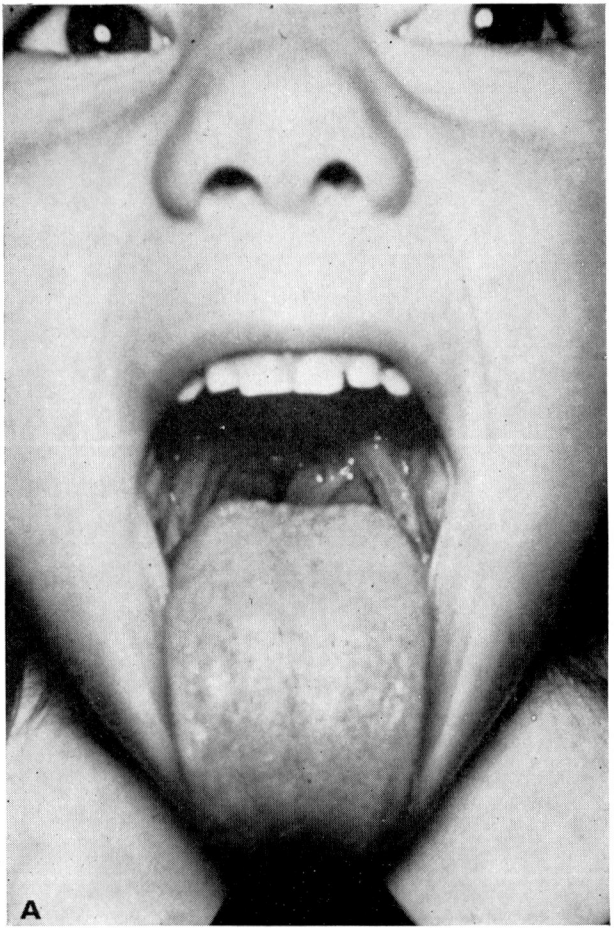

Figure 20A A, Size of tonsils can be deceptive: this child can by for-cibly protruding the tongue make the tonsils meet in the midline.

Figure 20B A tongue depressor if pressed on to the tongue causes 'gagging', which in this case results in the tonsils overlapping, B, whereas the tonsils are not conspicuous, C.

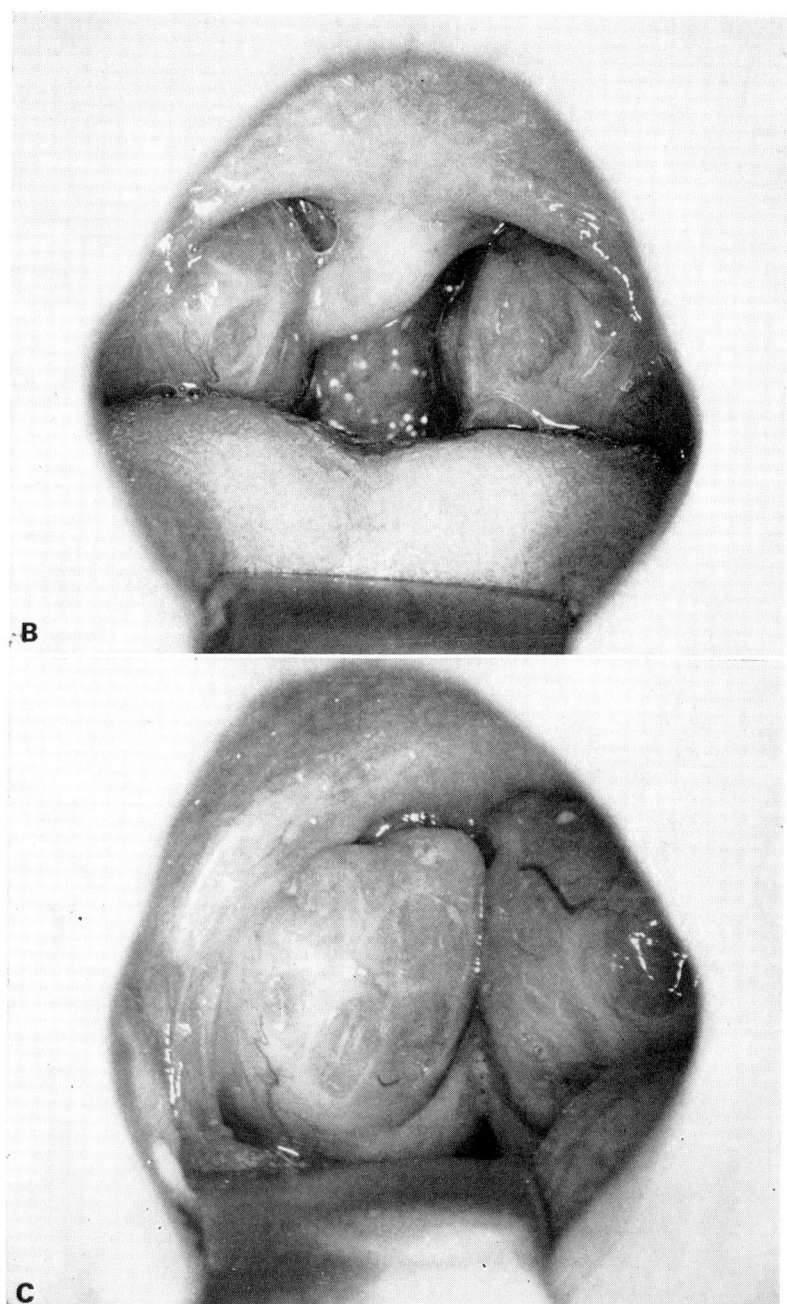

causing otitis media. The adenoids adjacent to the Eustachian orifice may be another factor underlying the otitis media, and the decision to remove adenoids, weighing the aural and possible speech problems, is therefore not easy. Removal of tonsils and adenoids is not an operation to be undertaken lightly, for although the complication of postoperative bleeding is uncommon it may occur and be serious. In a child under the age of five, the circulating blood volume is small, and a relatively small blood loss that would be of little consequence in an adult, may be serious to a small child. It is also emotionally disturbing for a child to come into hospital particularly for an operation that is followed by a painful throat, and sensible preparation and arrangements for the child by the parents, doctors and nurses and hospital administrators are necessary. For these reasons surgery is deferred when possible until the child is over four or five: the frequency of tonsillitis and the size of lymphoid tissue tend to regress after this age, which are further reasons for delay. When operation is necessary in younger children, it is often advisable for the mother to come into hospital with the child, and facilities for this are now available in many hospitals.

Parents are not infrequently extremely pressing in their desire for their children to have their tonsils and adenoids removed, and the reasons for delaying operation must be made clear to them, and also the limits of the operation: parents may think that many of their children's shortcomings, speech problems and unrelated symptoms stem from the tonsils and adenoids. A correct balance however is given by the ENT surgeon so that the child is not handicapped by an overconservative attitude to surgery.

Tonsillectomy in adult life carries less hazard than in children contrary to popular belief, and it is also dubious whether it is a more painful operation for an adult. After a quinsy, however, tonsillectomy is technically more difficult because dissection of the scar tissue deep to the tonsil involves more surgical trauma at the time of operation.

Nasal Obstruction

Whereas enlarged adenoids are the common cause of childhood nasal obstruction, there are many other causes for the common adult complaint of blocked nose. The voice with nasal obstruction lacks resonance and if the speech therapist detects poor resonance, an ENT opinion on the airway should be sought.

The bony and cartilaginous septum dividing the nostrils may be deviated or buckled in such a way to partially or totally obstruct both nasal fossae. A deviated septum is a common cause of nasal obstruction and is corrected by the operation of submucous resection (SMR). This is relatively minor nasal surgery in which the deviated portion of bone and cartilage is excised with preservation of the perichondrium and periostium on either side of the septum.

Nasal polypi are another common cause of nasal obstruction. Swelling of the nasal mucous membrane occurs in the ethmoid region and grey pendulous swellings form below the middle turbinate, which occlude the nasal fossae. These are benign lesions causing obstruction only, with no nose bleeding. They can be removed under local anaesthesia if they are small, but general anaesthesia is required for removal of extensive polypi.

Probably the commonest cause of nasal obstruction, however, is enlargement of the middle and inferior turbinates so that the mucous membrane may abut against the septum. This enlargement may be the result of allergy; in seasonal allergy, such as hay fever, this swelling is temporary, but when there are numerous allergic factors, a permanent swelling of the turbinates occurs. Turbinate enlargement may also result from long-standing irritation to the nasal mucous membrane. Tobacco, or dusty or dirty atmospheres are frequently responsible for this mucosal reaction. Nasal drops used to 'decongest' the nose during colds are, if used to excess, a common cause of turbinate enlargement and therefore such drops and sprays should only be used for a short period of time.

These types of 'irritative' enlargement of the turbinates are called chronic rhinitis and this is the condition frequently labelled by the patient as 'catarrh' or 'sinus trouble'. An excess of discharge of nasal mucous into the postnasal space is the complaint associated with the nasal obstruction. Chronic rhinitis is basically the response of a sensitive nasal mucous membrane to the environment and therefore, it is of course not always easy to treat or cure. If the turbinates are grossly enlarged, the airway can be improved by a surgical reduction in their size, and nasal cautery or diathermy to the turbinate mucous membrane is frequently used to achieve this.

Tongue-tie

Tongue-tie is a condition in which the attachment of short and tight frenulum extends to the tip of the tongue (Figure 21). The only obvious disability is an inability to protrude the tongue; this is commonly the only complaint and treatment is therefore unnecessary. The limitation of tongue

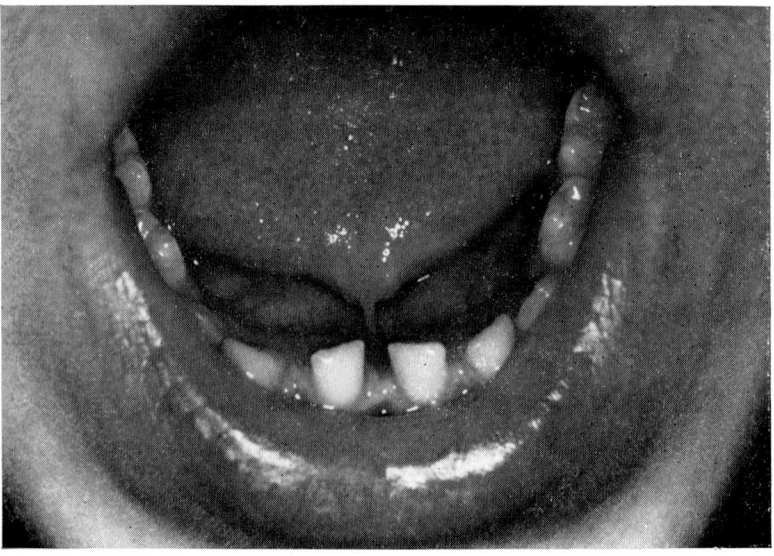

Figure 21   Tongue-tie. The frenulum linguae extends to the tip of the tongue and causes a 'pointed' appearance to the tongue.

movement may, however, on some occasions, alter the speech and surgical division of the frenulum may be necessary. Usually an incision and suturing to the frenulum is required under general anaesthesia; a 'snick' in an outpatient department is uncommonly adequate treatment. In the more severe cases there will be a history of some feeding difficulties in infancy and if the child is asked to protrude the tongue the characteristic notching of the tongue tip will be seen. The articulation of sound 'r' may sometimes be defective.

Parents may, if they are concerned with their child's speech development, inspect the tongue and suspect that a normal frenulum is limiting movement: reassurance is not uncommonly needed for this problem.

Globus Pharyngeus

A common throat symptom presented by patients in ENT clinics is the sensation of a lump, or a feeling of tightness or discomfort, in the region of the cricoid cartilage. This complaint is particularly common in those who are 'overaware' of their throat, commenting that they have a 'sensitive' or 'relaxed' throat; it tends to occur in the young anxious adult, and in those fearful of throat cancer. The onset may follow the knowledge of a friend or relation who has developed throat cancer. Patients with minor laryngeal pathology or psychogenic disorders are also susceptible to globus pharyngeus.

The sensation of a lump or throat 'tightness' is most noticeable when the patient swallows saliva. At mealtimes the symptom is absent. Although the condition is psychosomatic and perpetuated by worry and overattention to the throat, there is demonstrable spasm of the cricopharyngeus muscle often apparent on a barium swallow X-ray. The condition is also called globus hystericus, but this label may be misleading as the condition is not confined to hysterics, and may in fact be the presenting symptom of serious disease in the oesophagus or stomach. Globus pharyngeus, although usually only requiring reassurance and explanation as treatment, frequently calls for thorough investigation.

Deafness

The ear consists of three well-defined anatomical parts; the outer, middle and inner ear. The outer ear consists of the pinna and external auditory meatus which leads to the tympanic membrane or drum. The drum separates the meatus from the middle ear which is an air-filled cleft linked to the postnasal space by the Eustachian tube and containing the three ear ossicles, the malleus, incus and stapes. The footplate of the stapes bone forms a mobile joint at the oval window linking the middle to the inner ear. The drum and ossicles are mobile so that sound is transmitted from the outer to the inner ear. The inner ear contains the cochlea, which is stimulated by stapes movement and transmits impulses via the auditory nerve to the brain. The inner ear also contains three semicircular canals which are the main balance mechanisms of the body; it is not infrequent, therefore, for disorders of hearing to be associated with balance upsets, usually occurring as episodes of rotary unsteadiness or vertigo. Ménière's disease in which the vertigo is associated with an inner ear deafness and a ringing noise in the ears, tinnitus, is a common example of such an inner ear disease.

Deafness can be caused by obstruction of the external auditory meatus or by interference with the transmission of sound across the middle ear (Figure 22). Hearing loss caused by outer or middle ear disorders is called *conductive deafness* and this is frequently amenable to treatment. A conductive deafness will be caused, therefore, by such minor external ear conditions as impacted wax, or more serious obstruction such as congenital atresia of the meatus. A rigid or perforated tympanic membrane will also cause conductive deafness, as will any fixation or discontinuity of the ossicles. Bony fixation of the stapes in the oval window is a common cause of deafness in young and middle life, called otosclerosis. It is this condition that is frequently helped with a stapedectomy operation in which the immobile stapes bone is removed and replaced with a mobile teflon prosthesis. Secretory otitis media, in which the middle ear contains a sterile straw-coloured fluid, is another cause of conductive deafness. This condition may result from Eustachian tube obstruction occurring with a head cold or with barotrauma following flying; it is most common in children whose adenoids interfere with Eustachian tube function. A tenacious middle ear fluid accumulates ('glue ear') frequently making aspiration through an ear drum incision necessary (myringotomy). A teflon grommet ventilation tube is often inserted into the

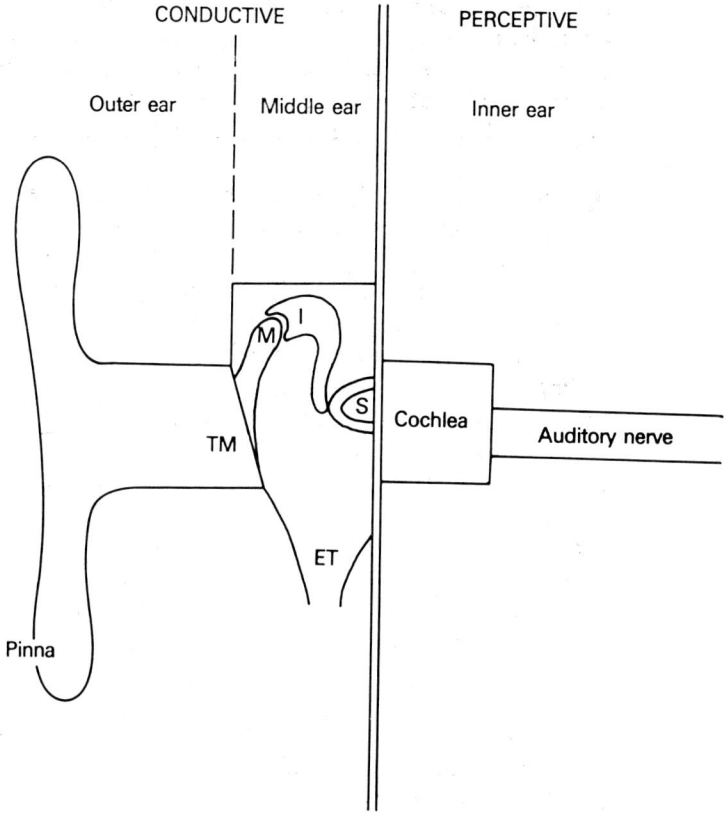

Figure 22   Types of deafness: diagrammatic description.

drum to maintain ventilation and an aerated middle ear. If the child's hearing has been affected for any length of time, the development of speech and language may be affected.

Damage or degeneration of the cochlea causes inner ear deafness, also called *perceptive or sensori-neural deafness*. Abnormal cochlear development, which may result from rubella (german measles) during pregnancy or a period of anoxia or severe jaundice soon after birth leads to congenital deafness; at the other end of the age scale, senile degeneration of the cochlea causes old age deafness, or presbycusis. Certain viruses may also damage the cochlea, and the mumps virus, particularly in adults, may cause total deafness in one ear. Exposure to noise, either as a single blast or prolonged intense noise, also causes sensori-neural deafness. Some drugs of which quinine, streptomycin, aspirin in excess doses are examples are known to damage the cochlea and are called ototoxic drugs. Unlike conductive deafness, perceptive deafness is rarely improved with treatment.

Lip reading The speech therapist may be asked to help an adult patient with an acquired hearing loss. If the hearing loss has been of gradual onset the patient may well have gained some ability in lip reading, although he may not be aware of this. Patients will say that they can hear better in a good light and if they face the speaker. This unconscious lip reading can be tested by covering the lower part of one's face while continuing to chat to the patient and noting whether they are able to follow as much of the conversation as hitherto. These patients do not need a full course of lip reading but can be helped to make their lip reading more efficient by better observation. Learning to interpret the various clues from facial expression, watching movements of the eyebrows, hands or shoulders are helpful, for example, the speaker when asking a question may raise his eyebrows and slightly lift the shoulders. They can also help themselves by being as widely read and conversant with current events as is possible, for they are then more likely to follow and understand when a news item is discussed.

If the hearing loss has been of more rapid onset it may be necessary to teach the patient to recognize the various consonant sounds, commencing with those most visible, p, b, m, and proceeding to those where there is no visible movement, k, g. As well as being able to recognize individual sounds help will be given so that phrases can be followed. The patient with a very sudden hearing loss will need help in adjusting to and accepting his disability.

The speech therapy for a deaf child or baby is a subject in itself and the management is often a long term undertaking and requires a specialized audiological unit.

CHAPTER SIX

CASE HISTORIES

Case histories of common speech disorders seen by speech therapists working with ENT surgeons are given as examples of some of the laryngeal conditions described in this book.

Mrs W Aged 48 Diagnosis: Vocal cord nodules

This lady presented with a hoarseness, which was worse in the morning or following prolonged talking. The diagnosis of vocal cord nodules was made by the ENT surgeon, who described these nodules, seen on indirect laryngoscopy, as small and symmetrical. The patient was referred to the speech therapist. The voice trouble had begun four months previously after lecturing at a training course. She had rested her voice for a short while, but had had to give a further series of lectures one month later. When the hoarseness persisted, she had sought advice.

The case history was taken which revealed that she had been under considerable strain for a long time. Her husband had had a severe coronary. He had been a difficult patient and refused to curtail or restrict his pattern of life in any form; he had died fifteen months previously. The patient had also been ill with bronchitis. She had had a long spell of sick leave and was concerned about her job.

Her voice sounded tired and 'breathy', and was produced with considerable effort. Breathing was clavicular, nasal resonance was limited and there was little attention to posture.

Treatment to achieve correct breathing and coordination of expiration and phonation was started and eventually progress was achieved.

Mrs W needed to talk over her problems, for she was concerned about her job and future, and also worried about her elderly mother who now lived with her. She was having difficulty in adjusting to being a widow. When the voice began to improve the stress over job future lessened, and she was finally given the appointment at work of investigating complaints. This gave her an opportunity of taking initiative, and her tact and ability to handle people was an asset. This gave her confidence, and her attitude made her new life easier.

Her voice has returned to normal, and when she was seen finally by the ENT surgeon, the vocal cord nodules were seen to have regressed, and direct microlaryngoscopy for removal of the nodules was not required.

Miss A J Aged 27 Diagnosis: Vocal cord nodules

This professional singer presented with hoarseness of three months duration. She was seen by the ENT surgeon and the diagnosis of moderately large singer's nodules was made: she was referred for speech therapy.

Miss A J was working with a very successful pop-group, and had the pressure of heavy singing commitments with little time to rest. On many occasions she was singing in smokey and dusty atmospheres where the amplification for the group was not adequate, and she felt compelled to 'force' her voice. In addition she had recently had to sing with a cold. Following this episode, she has developed hoarseness which was not only apparent in her speaking voice, but was limiting and prejudicing her singing performance. The group have several future engagements and although the ENT surgeon had advised a two week period of rest at first, pending speech therapy, Miss A J was extremely pressing to get back to work. The patient was very keen to improve her method of voice production and was understandably anxious for quick results rather than prolonged treatment. It was difficult in these circumstances to arrange appointments on a regular basis following a period of voice rest. Some advice on correct and more relaxed voice production was given and this patient's voice returned to near normal, and she was able to continue with her work.

Miss A J was again seen six weeks following her initial visit by the ENT surgeon, and the nodules were still present.

The routine of heavy bookings, late and long hours working and much travelling, was the typical history of a successful singer, and although her voice remained adequate, a correct period of voice rest and treatment was never achieved and persistent hoarseness developed. The nodules became larger and well established, and surgical removal followed by speech therapy and time off work was advised.

Master K F   Aged 15   Diagnosis: Screamer's nodules

This boy presented with a history of hoarseness over four months. He was seen by the ENT surgeon, and the diagnosis of screamer's nodules was made. In view of the size of the nodules and the degree of hoarseness surgery was advised. The speech therapist was asked to see the patient in order to assess the voice prior to surgery. The father accompanied the boy for his speech therapy assessment. There did not appear to be excessive voice use at home, but there was a history of enthusiastic shouting whilst playing football or watching it. There was a long history of mouth-breathing, this was confirmed by observation although a normal nasal airway was noted at the ENT examination. There was also the expected shallow clavicular breathing and an absence of any degree of nasal resonance. The boy demonstrated, when requested, that nose-breathing was possible. He was given exercises to help establish normal nose-breathing and to promote better lip closure. Work was also given to obtain correct diaphragmatic breathing. The voice work however in this case was not commenced until after surgical removal of the nodules.

Mrs S   Aged 52   Diagnosis: Chronic laryngitis

This patient with hoarseness was seen at indirect laryngoscopy by the ENT surgeon to have polypoid margins of the vocal cords. A speech therapy opinion was requested about the method of voice production.

The patient complained that prolonged talking was tiring and produced a feeling of discomfort in her throat. On discussing her voice problem she said her father had had increasing deafness for many years and the whole family shouted to make him hear. She had a part-time voluntary job which did not involve much talking and she felt she was a moderate talker in social situations. There was a history of increasing breathlessness on exertion, particularly for the last two years. Her breathing however seemed to be diaphragmatic. The voice lacked any nasal resonance, and if she tried to achieve volume, there was visible neck forcing. It was felt that these vocal habits were so well established that speech therapy alone would achieve little improvement in the voice. The patient was admitted for microlaryngoscopy and the polypoid margin of the vocal cords were excised leaving the mucosa of the anterior portion of the less oedematous cord.

There was an immediate improvement in the voice following operation, and the patient was referred for speech therapy. Exercises to the neck and shoulders and breathing were started. She had practised yoga and so found the breathing exercises very easy. Nasal resonance was improved to help give volume to the voice. She was seen twice, and then went on holiday; when she returned, good voice production was established; she found she could cope even if there was background noise and there was no feeling of discomfort in the throat or neck.

Mr C Aged 72 Diagnosis: Carcinoma of left vocal cord; Laryngofissure

This man presented with a history of hoarseness for four years. He was seen by the ENT surgeon, first as an outpatient, and he was admitted for microlaryngoscopy. At this investigation, a biopsy was taken, and the pathologist's report confirmed the diagnosis of carcinoma of the left vocal cord. Mr C was then referred to the radiotherapist, and underwent a full course of radiotherapy. He remained free of disease for about seven months when a further laryngeal biopsy revealed a recurrence of carcinoma. He underwent a laryngofissure operation. His voice postoperatively was breathy due to an escape at the site of the excised vocal cord, and he relied on a forced whisper for conversation. There was considerable strain involved to produce this whisper. Expiration was not coordinated with attempts at phonation.

Work was begun on glottal attack, breathing exercises and resonance. He was a cooperative patient and quickly grasped the idea of expiration of air when phonating, and that in view of air waste it was necessary to keep replenishing the air supply. In view of the travelling involved, he was only seen twice by the speech therapist, but during these visits, he had gained sufficient knowledge to use his altered vocal mechanism to best advantage.

Mr B   Aged 28   Diagnosis: Vocal cord palsy (idiopathic)

An actor had developed voice difficulties while working in a Christmas show. His main complaint was of a 'weak' voice. He was initially treated for laryngitis with antibiotics and inhalations, and he continued in the show, but after three weeks, his voice started fading, and eventually became almost inaudible. ENT examination showed a right cord palsy. All investigations showed no apparent cause for this. The diagnosis was made of an idiopathic right cord palsy. (It is more common for the left to be involved.)

When he first attended for speech therapy, he had been away from work for two and a half weeks and was concerned about future bookings. He had the typical, fading 'breathy' voice of vocal cord paresis. His motivation to cooperate was high, and his knowledge of voice production helped this patient in spite of his understandable concern regarding his future.

Work on glottal attack and breathing exercises was started. When these were well established, resonance exercises were begun. He then insisted on returning to rehearsals against advice and coped well, until during one performance he felt his voice begin to fade and panicked. This increased general tension and so altered his breathing which became quick and shallow. This unfortunate experience persuaded him to stop acting for a time, and so give himself more chance of achieving better vocal cord compensation. Six months after the onset of the hoarseness, indirect laryngoscopy showed some return of vocal cord movement, and at nine months, a normal voice, with full movement of the right cord, had returned.

A teflon injection to the larynx had been considered for this patient, and he was putting considerable pressure on both the ENT surgeon and speech therapist, to obtain a normal voice rapidly. Spontaneous recovery or full compensation is however not infrequent with idiopathic vocal cord palsy, and patience and surgical conservatism was rewarded.

Christopher W Aged 12 Diagnosis: Vocal cord palsy

This boy underwent thoracic surgery for repair of a patent ductus arteriosus seven months before being seen by the ENT surgeon complaining of hoarseness. A left vocal cord palsy was diagnosed as a complication of his thoracic surgery. There was little compensation by the right vocal cord, and there was considerable air escape on phonation, due to failure of full adduction of the cords. He was referred to the speech therapy department.

The thoracic surgeon was satisfied with the surgical result, but the mother had noticed that Christopher's voice had altered; it was hoarse and he seemed unable to cough normally, and he had a peculiar laugh. Christopher was very apprehensive that he might need further surgery, and was an inveterate worrier.

His voice was forced and had the characteristic 'breathy' quality of a cord palsy; it was also slightly higher than normal in pitch.

Glottal exercises were given, and Christopher was made aware of the need to breathe in at frequent intervals; he was encouraged to achieve quieter and easier breath taking. He was soon able to produce good glottal sounds and the voice became less 'breathy'. Later exercises to improve resonance and volume were given. When reviewed again a year later, he had a clear, normal voice. Indirect laryngoscopy showed the left cord palsy to be permanent, but there was good compensation by the right cord and on phonation, there was little air escape.

Miss F Aged 19 Diagnosis: Functional aphonia

This young lady was already attending the ENT outpatient department for a series of minor complaints: she arrived one day totally aphonic. She was a supply teacher, and had been teaching in a difficult school during a heat wave. The children had been disorderly and finally she had slapped a child. This resulted in a severe warning from the school inspector that she would lose her job if this occurred again. She was not allowed to work the following day, and after the weekend, started at another school. She began to notice voice difficulties, and within two days, she was unable to speak above a whisper. ENT examination showed a normal larynx, but with failure to maintain adduction on phonation.

This girl had innumerable problems. She was an epileptic, although this was fairly well controlled by drugs. She had frequent colds and sinusitis. She had come to this country from abroad three years ago, and while she wanted to stay here, she also felt she should return to visit her family. She hated teaching. Her views on life and morals were somewhat confused and generally seemed to add to her agitated state. She coughed very loudly at frequent intervals.

Work on gentle breathing and resonance was started, and she was able to produce some voice. By the following visit, her voice was nearly normal but there was still some forcing. Indirect laryngoscopy showed no abnormality. She had by now decided to return home in about five months, and was advised to think of a future career other than teaching. It was suggested that she took a secretarial course so that she could earn some money and give herself time to decide on a career. Speech therapy was not continued.

Mrs J   Aged 28   Diagnosis: Functional dysphonia

This lady presented to the ENT surgeon with a history of a 'peculiar voice' for five weeks, which had developed during an attack of influenza. She complained that her throat felt tight and uncomfortable. Despite a curious and gross hoarseness, indirect laryngoscopy, which was difficult because the patient found the examination unpleasant, showed a completely normal larynx. A functional voice problem was therefore diagnosed, and the patient referred for speech therapy.

The patient worked as a secretary, and her husband was employed in the same company as a business executive. Her job involved a certain amount of talking, but the conditions were fairly quiet. She had had some stress throughout the preceding year. Her divorce had come through exactly a year ago, and there had been difficulties with this. She had then become engaged and shortly afterwards, her future mother-in-law and sister-in-law had come over for a visit from abroad. While she had found her mother-in-law pleasant, the sister-in-law was moody and difficult, following a broken engagement. Mrs J had remarried 4 months previously, and had continued her full time job. She and her husband planned to go abroad in about a year's time. They would not start a family until the new business was established. She was fully in agreement with this plan, but she wanted a family soon. We discussed this at some length, for whilst she agreed with the logic of their future plans, her own wishes were different. It was suggested that she and her husband should discuss this and she should make him fully aware of her wishes.

In listening to Mrs J's voice, one noted mouth-breathing, shallow clavicular breathing, and a forced harsh voice. Voice exercises were started and at the next visit she had a nearly normal voice. She had decided to work part-time only. At the third visit, her voice was completely normal. Shortly after this, her husband was offered a senior post in the company, so they remained in this country, and a year later she gave birth to a daughter.

Miss T W   Aged 14   Diagnosis: Functional aphonia

This young girl presented with a loss of voice and sore throat following a cold. She was seen by the ENT surgeon, and on examination the larynx was found to be normal. The diagnosis of functional aphonia was made, and the girl was referred for speech therapy.

A full case history was taken, but this revealed no possible causes of strain or stress. She had been a weekly boarder at school for about nine months, and her mother admitted that there had been some stress at settling in to a new routine, but that this now seemed to have been accepted and Tessa had settled at school. She appeared to have plenty of friends and many interests. Apparently the school was fairly rigid regarding illness, and as soon as a girl reported sick, she was sent to sick-bay. Tessa had been somewhat upset by having a cold and sore throat and then being isolated in sick bay, and one could only conclude that a temporary loss of voice due to infection had been perpetuated by isolation in sick-bay, and worry as to a possible serious cause. Her alarm had no doubt been increased by being sent home. She was reassured by the ENT surgeon that there was no infection.

Gentle voice exercises were started and sounds were heard. This encouraged Tessa who felt a normal voice was likely to be achieved. She was allowed to return to school for the last few days of term, when normal voice returned.

Miss S P Aged 16 Diagnosis: Functional dysphonia

This adolescent presented with a history of hoarseness for seven weeks. She was seen by the ENT surgeon who was unable to obtain a clear view of the larynx with indirect laryngoscopy, and she was admitted for direct laryngoscopy: the larynx was found to be normal. The diagnosis of functional dysphonia was made. She had a very bizarre voice and was referred for a tape recording to be taken in the first instance, to be followed by speech therapy. The father however, removed the child from hospital and would not allow any further treatment.

The patient reappeared two years later with the same curious hoarse voice and this time she attended for speech therapy and a proper case history was taken. It appeared that her parents had divorced when she was three years old and she had lived with her father. She went abroad with her father at frequent intervals. When she was of school age, she had several different tutors and teachers who travelled with her and her father. Shortly after the first attack of hoarseness she left her father and went to live with her mother. She was often left to run the home and look after her young brother whilst her mother was abroad on business. She was not mature enough to cope with the responsibility. It would seem that her father had removed Sally from treatment so that a full investigation of possible contributory factors could not be undertaken. Whilst this girl had numerous problems, her voice responded well to speech therapy, reassurance and the opportunity to talk over her problems.

Mr H R Aged 64 Laryngectomy

This man presented with a history of hoarseness for approximately four months. He also complained of a mild sore throat. Indirect laryngoscopy revealed a lesion on the left ventricular band. He was admitted for microlaryngoscopy when a supraglottic tumour was found. A biopsy was taken and the report showed squamous cell carcinoma. He was referred for radiotherapy and underwent a full course. Further microlaryngoscopy and biopsy showed residual disease and the patient was prepared for laryngectomy. He was apprehensive as a brother had a laryngectomy twenty years ago. The brother never acquired a pseudo-voice and died of pneumonia some months after surgery. The speech therapist was asked to see the patient preoperatively. Two visits were made in view of the patient's apprehension. A brief explanation of the new voice mechanism was given each time and the patient reassured. The wife was present one visit and she wanted to know why a mechanical voice box could not be fitted in at the time of surgery. She did not seem able to give her husband any support.

Following surgery Mr R made an uneventful recovery. Voice work was started two and a half weeks after surgery. Noise was achieved. He was extremely agitated and easily confused. He received no reassurance and help from his wife. He was discharged home—still somewhat tense and depressed. His wife refused to help him manage his stoma. She refused even to watch and made no effort to understand his mouthings or attempts at voicing. In spite of this the patient has acquired pseudo-voice. He is now well able to converse during his daily visits to the local pub.

It would seem the slow start in acquiring pseudo-voice was due in part to the rather tense home situation and the lack of assistance from his wife.

INDEX